The Essential Guide To

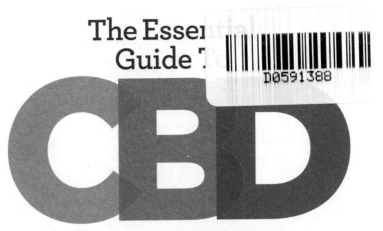

CBD

EVERYTHING YOU NEED TO KNOW
ABOUT WHAT IT HELPS, WHERE TO BUY,
AND HOW TO TAKE IT

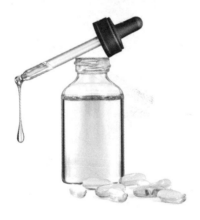

Editors of Reader's Digest and Project CBD

Reader's
Digest

Reader's Digest
New York • Montreal

Images copyright Shutterstock: cover (2), pp. 4, 9, 10-11, 13 (2), 14 (2), 20 (2), 26, 27, 43, 50, 52, 56, 58, 61, 62-63, 65, 66, 69, 75, 81, 83 (2), 87, 90, 95, 109, 115, 117, 121, 124, 128, 132-133, 142, 151, 152, 154, 164, 187, 191, 202, 206, 227, 232; George McKeon: pp. 16, 30, 36, 161, 178; Joleen Zubek: pp. 28, 123, 163; Courtesy Michelle Smith: p. 34; Joseph Siciliano/Courtesy Greg Gerdeman: p. 42; Courtesy DEFY: p. 49; Courtesy Emily Wilson: p. 71; Steve Vaccariello and Bryan Christie: pp. 76, 104, 110; Joel Silva/Courtesy Bonni Goldstein: p. 80; Matt Nager: p. 84; Courtesy Greenwich Biosciences: p. 99; Courtesy Damaris Higuera: p. 100; Michael Kozart/Courtesy Melina Misuraca: p. 102; Jamie Livingood Photography/Courtesy Selene Yeager: p. 106; Courtesy VJVONART: p. 111; Sam Gehrke Photography/Courtesy Janelle Lassalle: p. 118; Rachel Hinman for Highland Pantry/Courtesy Aliza Sherman Risdahl: p. 130; Courtesy Project CBD: p. 138; Courtesy Precision Extraction Solutions: p. 139; Courtesy N.B. Oler Engineering: p. 140; Russell Porcas: pp. 141, 214, 218, 222, 224; Courtesy Alex Malkin: p. 155; Robert McMillan/Courtesy Patricia McMillan: p. 180; Courtesy Jahan Marcu: p. 190; Mark Gordon Murray/Courtesy Anna Symonds: p. 199; Kelly Dobrowolski/Courtesy Michael Dobrowolski: p. 229

NOTE TO OUR READERS

The information in this book should not be substituted for, or used to alter, medical therapy without your doctor's advice. For a specific health problem, consult your physician for guidance.

Mention of specific companies, organizations, or authorities in this book does not imply endorsement by the author or publisher, nor does mention of specific companies, organizations, or authorities imply that they endorse this book, its author, or the publisher. The brand-name products mentioned in this book are trademarks or registered trademarks of their respective companies. Internet addresses and telephone numbers given in this book were accurate at the time it went to press.

Acknowledgments

Many thanks to Project CBD co-founder and director Martin A. Lee, whose vision, expertise, and passion shaped this book from the beginning. Special thanks also go to Project CBD contributors Tiffany Devitt, Adrian Devitt-Lee, Quinn Supplee, Sara Alsop, Zoe Sigman, Daphne Church, Alana Lee, Anna Symonds, Melinda Misuraca, Mary Biles, Greg Gerdeman, Gary Richter, Nishi Whitely, Bonni Goldstein, Dustin Sulak, Stacey Kerr, Viola Brugnatelli, Jahan Marcu, and Sarah Russo.

At Reader's Digest and its parent company, Trusted Media Brands, the following were key champions of the book: Bruce Kelley, chief content officer; Jeremy Greenfield, senior editor, new product development; Courtney Murphy, creative director; Rebecca Steele, visuals director; Nancy Taylor, director, trade specialty markets; Christi Crowley, director of sales, trade publishing; and Andrea Levitt, senior editor, books.

Selene Yeager, writer extraordinaire, went above and beyond the call of duty to make sense of the profusion of information (and misinformation) about CBD. Melinda Misuraca developed the recipes, while Russell Porcas photographed them. And George McKeon, art director, pulled it all together.

Finally, Project CBD and Reader's Digest are grateful to the people who courageously shared their personal stories in this book: Laura Dobratz, Michael Dobrowolski, Terrell Davis, Brian and Sadie Higuera, Stephanie Johnson, Josh Kincaid, Janelle Lassalle, Alex Malkin, Laurie Maxson, Patricia McMillan, Melinda Misuraca, Aliza Sherman Risdahl, Michelle Smith, Anna Symonds, VJ Von Art, Emily Wilson, and Selene Yeager.

CONTENTS

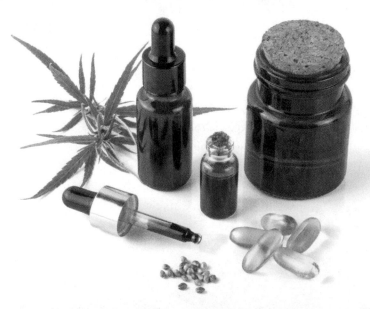

The CBD Revolution

I F YOU FEEL like you'd never heard of CBD just a few years ago and now you can't go a week without hearing about this "new miracle cure-all," you're not alone.

The big tipping point came between 2014 and 2018, when under increased public demand to decriminalize cannabis, Congress passed Farm Bills that changed the way hemp could be grown and sold. Specifically, the bills included a qualification that cannabis can be considered hemp and not marijuana as long as the plant contains no more than 0.3 percent tetrahydrocannabinol (THC), the chemical in marijuana that gets you high.[1] This effectively made it legal to grow and presumably also to sell and consume hemp-based CBD products.

And the marketplace exploded. The sale of CBD products skyrocketed 706 percent from the passage of the second Farm Bill in 2018 to the end of 2019. The research firm Brightfield Group estimates that, by 2023, the total U.S. CBD market could reach $23.7 billion.[2]

These days you can buy CBD coffee, face creams, shampoo, deodorant, bath bombs, tinctures, gummies, sparkling water, iced tea, soda, vape cartridges, chocolate bars, dog treats, soft gels, lotions, sports drinks, protein powders, suppositories, patches, eye drops, and supposedly even CBD-infused pillows, mattresses, and athletic wear. And we've probably missed a few.

Though CBD (as the pharmaceutical drug Epidiolex) is only officially FDA approved for the treatment of pediatric seizure disorders, it has acquired a reputation as a cure-all that's good for preventing or treating a very long list of health and wellness issues, including sleep disturbances, anxiety, pain, inflammation, brain injuries, menopausal symptoms, weight loss, heart disease, cancer, Parkinson's disease, depression, stress, multiple sclerosis, addiction, eczema, acne, diabetes, GI disorders, and much, much more.

> Scientists are working hard to understand how CBD works.

Could one substance possibly help treat all these things? Is it safe to use? And where do you start if you're ready to try it? You'll find the answers to these and many other questions about CBD in this practical guide.

The current body of clinical research is relatively small because the federal government has been slow to support investigations into the therapeutic potential of CBD and other cannabis compounds. Now, in many countries around the world, scientists are working hard to understand how CBD works, how it affects the brain, and how it can improve our health. But these studies take time. As we have for almost 100 years, the editors at Reader's Digest have read through much of the relevant medical literature and talked to the top experts in the field—along with readers like you, who have tried CBD—to get the facts for you.

In Part I of the book, we'll lay out the basics of what CBD is and how it works. We'll also tackle some common misconceptions about CBD.

In Part II, we'll examine in more detail how CBD may be helpful against more than 30 common health conditions, from anxiety to cancer to weight issues, complete with the scientific evidence that currently exists.

In Part III, you'll learn how to pick the type of product that will work best for your needs. (Some conditions respond best when you take CBD orally, while others do just fine with a topical treatment.) We'll help you find your sweet spot for dosing (large doses can have the opposite effect of small doses) while avoiding side effects, including potentially serious drug interactions.

We'll also show you how to navigate the marketplace, which is full of shoddy products and outright fraud. Penn Medicine researchers found that nearly 70 percent of CBD products they purchased online were incorrectly labeled and contained either more or less cannabidiol than the label indicated. More than 20 percent of the products also contained THC.[3] Many people are mistakenly buying hemp seed oil, which has zero CBD. We'll tell you what you need to know to find high-quality products you can trust.

You'll even find special sections on CBD for pets and recipes for making your own CBD products. Plus, throughout the book, people who have tried different types of CBD for a variety of health issues share their experience and advice.

To help pull this all together, Reader's Digest has partnered with Project CBD, a California-based nonprofit dedicated to promoting and publicizing research into the medical uses of cannabidiol (CBD) and other components of the cannabis plant. Established in 2010 by journalists who had been covering the medical marijuana story, Project CBD was instrumental in introducing CBD to the medical cannabis community in California, and it spread from there. Project CBD provides educational services for physicians, patients, industry professionals, and the general public.

As part of their mission, Project CBD updates doctors and patients on developments in cannabis science, therapeutics, and political economy. They support the efforts of physicians and other researchers to collect, aggregate, and publish data from people using cannabidiol for medical reasons to determine patterns of CBD efficacy—or lack of efficacy. They conduct training workshops for

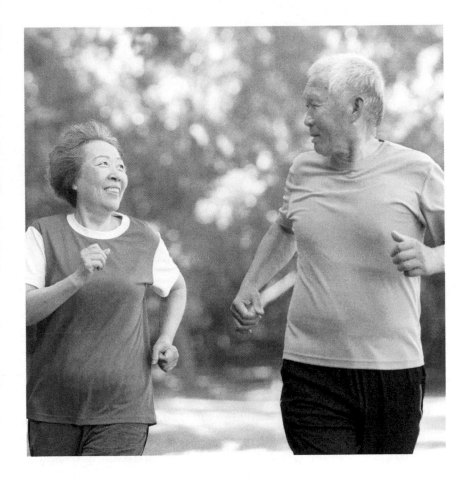

consumers, health workers, and dispensary staff on the benefits and challenges of CBD-rich therapeutics. And they help people navigate this complicated landscape and find high-quality CBD-rich medicine.

It is indeed a very confusing time to be a CBD consumer. Right now there is fascinating science, promising evidence, and a lot of unknowns. Together, Reader's Digest and Project CBD will separate fact from fiction, hype from reality, so you and your family can best tap into the promise of CBD to improve your health and wellness.

1

CBD Basics

"I T SOUNDS TOO good to be true."

That's how a lot of people respond when they hear the long list of benefits CBD can have on their physical and mental well-being. After all, what kind of supplement can kill pain, lower blood pressure, fight dementia, improve sleep, and promote weight loss, just to name a few?

Well, CBD isn't just a "supplement" like a vitamin C or calcium pill. It is a molecule that actually mimics and helps support the innate health and wellness regulating system within your body: the endocannabinoid system (ECS). The ECS is involved in nearly every single biological process, including digestion, metabolism, hormone regulation, appetite, immunity, memory, emotions, sleep, and much more.

Scientists discovered the endocannabinoid system when they were trying to understand how cannabis works; instead they discovered a cellular gold mine of information about how we work.

It turns out we are literally wired to respond to cannabinoid compounds that interact with receptors in our brain, nervous system, immune system, organs, even our skin. And we naturally make our own cannabinoids—known as endocannabinoids—to keep this system humming along. But we also can fortify our endocannabinoid system, support it, and optimize it—along with our health—by consuming plant-derived cannabinoids, like CBD, one of the many cannabinoids found in the cannabis plant.

So, yes, CBD really is that good. But it's not necessarily simple. There is a great deal of information—and misinformation—about this mighty molecule. So this section provides a detailed look at what CBD is and how it works in your body.

You'll learn where CBD comes from, how it interacts with other plant-derived and endogenous cannabinoids, and why it is essential to choose products that are made from the right kinds of plants.

You'll also take a journey through the endocannabinoid system, complete with a deep dive into its many roles as a master regulator of your basic human functions, as well as an antioxidant, an anti-inflammatory, a brain cell builder, and mood manager. You'll also learn how this essential system can become dysfunctional through stress, sedentary living, and poor nutrition, like that found in the Standard American Diet. Endocannabinoid dysfunction, it turns out, underlies nearly every disease known to human beings.

This section will answer the questions you may have on why the CBD market is so confusing and why, though scientists around the world have discovered dozens of medical benefits, CBD manufacturers are still undergoing federal and legal battles because of antiquated marijuana laws.

Finally, this section will clearly dispel myths and separate fact from fiction when it comes to cannabis-based preparations that include CBD, as well as its more maligned cousin cannabinoid, tetrahydrocannabinol (THC), which is best known for causing a "high" but can also play an important role in health and wellness.

By the time you turn the final page of Part I, it'll be abundantly clear why CBD has become so wildly popular and you'll have a comprehensive understanding of where it comes from, how it can work for you, and why it really isn't "too good to be true."

1

What Is CBD?

T HE WAY CBD has been splashed across the nation's headlines, taken the country by storm, and had many companies considering adding this new "miracle supplement" to their drinks, you'd think it was some brand-new chemical cure-all cooked up in a 21st-century laboratory.

Actually, CBD, which is short for cannabidiol, is anything but new. CBD is a naturally occurring compound extracted from cannabis plants. Although we "discovered" the CBD molecule relatively recently, the cannabis plant it comes from has been with us and has been used medicinally for thousands of years. It has a broad range of actions including reducing anxiety, inflammation, and stress, among other myriad health benefits.

Cannabis: "A Medicinal Treasure Trove"

Cannabis has been part of the *pharmacopeia*, or branch of medical science that studies drugs and medicinal preparations, of many cultures throughout history.

Like many other plants, cannabis plants secrete a sticky tar-like residue called resin. On cannabis plants, the resin is contained within the heads of tiny, mushroom-shaped trichomes, found mainly on the plant's flower buds and to a lesser extent on the leaves. In the *resin* is tetrahydrocannabinol (THC)—the compound that causes the high that cannabis is famous for—and CBD, along with hundreds of other cannabinoids and terpenes (which we'll talk about later). Traditionally, these flowers, which we commonly call marijuana, are hand-harvested, dried, trimmed, and cured. The flowers are then consumed for their medicinal and/or intoxicating effects.

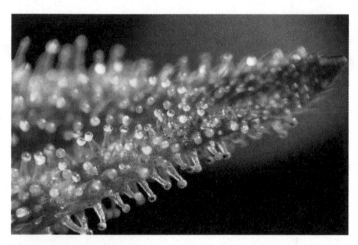

Trichomes on flowers and leaves

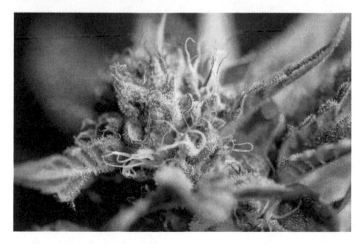

Marijuana flowers on the plant

Israeli scientist Raphael Mechoulam, one of the world's leading authorities on CBD, has described the cannabis plant as a "treasure trove" of medicinal value with the potential to treat a wide variety of different ailments. CBD and THC can be considered the crown

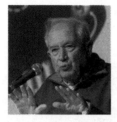

jewels of this treasure trove, but they are just two of more than a hundred related plant compounds called *phytocannabinoids*, lipid (fat)-based molecules that are unique to the cannabis plant and give it its therapeutic potential. The plant is also rich in compounds called *terpenes* and *flavonoids*,

Raphael Mechoulam   which work together with CBD and THC to create

Plant Cannabinoids

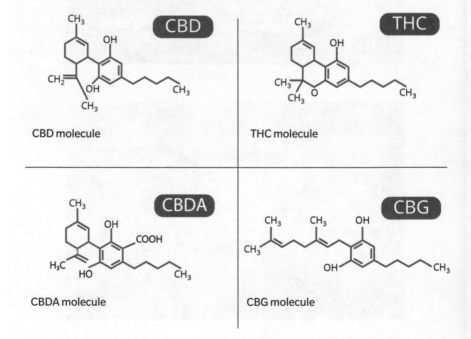

CBD molecule

THC molecule

CBDA molecule

CBG molecule

an "entourage effect" that is greater than the effect of any one of the molecules alone.

CBD is getting the lion's share of public attention right now because, unlike THC, it doesn't get you high or put you at risk for failing a drug test; nor is it likely to pose legal challenges like THC. It's important to bear in mind, though, that CBD is not the only part of the cannabis plant that can serve a medicinal purpose.

CBD and Its Entourage

CBD and THC have a bit of a yin-yang relationship. Both CBD and THC can provide significant health and wellness benefits; but unlike THC, CBD does not make a person feel "stoned." That's because CBD and THC act in different ways on different receptors in the brain and body.

THC, marijuana's principal psychoactive component, makes a person feel high by binding to specific receptors in your brain and central nervous system. (Chapter 2 will dive into these mechanisms in detail). CBD, by contrast, can lessen or neutralize the intoxicating effects of THC, depending on how much of each compound is consumed. That's why people who use medical marijuana will sometimes choose products that are relatively low in THC and rich in CBD. They want the health benefits of cannabis without the high—or with less of the high. That's possible, thanks to CBD.

There is compelling evidence that CBD works best in combination with THC and the full spectrum of other cannabis components. Just like eating a whole carrot is better for you than taking a beta-carotene supplement, whole cannabis remedies may be more effective than low-THC or no-THC products.

That's important as we consider the medicinal benefits of CBD (and when you're choosing CBD products) because, when scientists perform research on CBD, they generally use isolated, single-molecule CBD produced in biochemical laboratories. By contrast,

The State of Legal Cannabis

Right now, cannabis is legal in some capacity in the majority of the United States, and CBD and THC are legal as a prescribed pharmaceutical under federal law.[1] CBD is also legal if it's present in or extracted from "hemp," a cannabis plant with 0.3 percent THC (or less), whereas CBD—the same substance—is illegal if it comes from a cannabis plant with more than 0.3 percent THC. Depending on where you live, it is entirely possible at this time to be using a cannabis-based product in accordance with your state's laws while simultaneously violating the federal law.

The disconnect can be found right in our U.S. Constitution. The Tenth Amendment of the Constitution generally delegates police powers to the states. That means if you live in Colorado, for example, where marijuana is legal for both recreational and medicinal use, the state cannot prosecute you (if you're 21 or older) for using the drug, but the federal government still can.

Though it's increasingly less likely that the federal government will bring charges to individuals in any given state for personal cannabis use, ongoing federal prohibition makes it very difficult for scientists at universities to receive federal grants to study cannabis and its components.

The following map reflects the legal status of CBD and cannabis in the United States at this time. The laws are changing quickly, however, so check https://norml.org/ for the most up-to-date status of CBD and cannabis laws in your state and on the federal level.

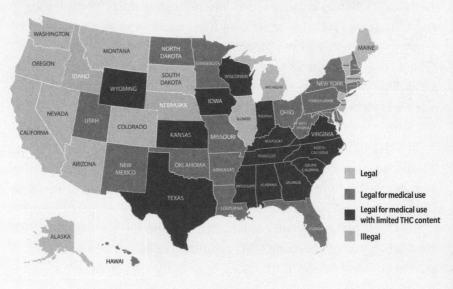

when CBD is part of oil extracted from the whole plant, it includes not just CBD and THC but also more than 400 trace compounds, many of which may also have medicinal benefits. In fact, as this book is being written, scientists are turning their attention to other CBD-related molecules that have exciting therapeutic potential—for example, CBDA and CBG. CBDA is the acidic, raw form of CBD that exists in the growing CBD-rich plant before it has been harvested, dried, and heated and may be even more effective against nausea than CBD or THC.[2] Cannabigerol (CBG) is another cannabinoid that has medicinal value as an analgesic, anti-inflammatory, antidepressant, bone stimulant, and cancer-fighting molecule.[3]

Researchers have found that many of these compounds interact synergistically to create an "entourage effect" or "ensemble effect." In the same way that a star opera singer sounds great on her own but creates a greater impact as part of a cast of supporting singers, these myriad compounds magnify the benefits of the plant's individual components so that the medicinal impact of the whole plant is greater than the sum of its parts.

Some of the key "backup singers" in that entourage are *terpenes*. Terpenes are aromatic molecules that evaporate easily and create a strong fragrance. You may not know their names, but you already know these compounds because they're ingrained in your life. The fresh scent of lemon zest is from the terpene limonene. The refreshing aroma wafting through a pine forest comes from the terpene aptly named pinene.

Terpenes are the most common type of compound in the botanical world; there are hundreds of terpenes among all the cannabis strains, and there can be 20 to 40 types of terpenes in a single cannabis plant. The fragrance and flavor of any given cannabis product is determined by its predominant terpenes. Nature designed these pungent oils to protect plants by attracting beneficial insects, or by repelling harmful ones and animal grazers, as well as preventing damaging fungus.

It turns out terpenes are healthy for people as well as plants.

Pinene, which is found not only in the oils of pine and other conif-erous trees but also in rosemary, is known for its anti-inflammatory effects.[4] *Beta-caryophyllene*, a terpene found in black pepper, oregano, leafy green vegetables, and various cannabis strains may be good for treating certain ulcers and auto-immune disorders. Linalool, the dominant terpene from lavender, alters brain wave activity and pro-motes relaxation.[5]

Some terpene compounds (called terpenoids) increase blood flow. Others enhance brain activity and kill germs, including MRSA, the antibiotic-resistant bacteria that have claimed the lives of tens of thousands of Americans. An article published in the *British Journal of Pharmacology* reports the findings from multiple studies showing that cannabinoid-terpenoid interactions—that entourage effect—could work well for more effective treatment of pain, inflammation, depression, anxiety, addiction, epilepsy, cancer, and infections.[6]

In various ways, terpenes can augment the beneficial effects of CBD and THC. Research shows that terpenes can help cannabinoids like CBD and THC cross the blood-brain barrier and get into your system more easily.[7] Some terpenes may facilitate transdermal absorption to allow topical treatments to pass through the skin.

It's important to keep this entourage effect in mind when reading the results of scientific studies. When a study reports that a certain dosage of CBD did not have an effect, that doesn't necessarily mean that CBD doesn't work. Any given dose of single-molecule CBD is not medicinally the same as the same dose of a CBD-rich whole plant can-nabis extract.[8] Often, you actually need considerably higher doses of an isolated CBD product to get the same benefits you'd find from a smaller amount of whole plant CBD extract because of the entourage effect.

CBD and Cannabis Confusion

If CBD is so good for us and has been around for thousands of years, why are we just hearing about it now? The short answer is because

A Brief History of Cannabis in Medicine

Cannabis originally evolved in Asia, where it was used as herbal medicine at least as early as 2700 B.C., according to historians. From there it spread to the Middle East, Africa, Europe, and the Americas.[9]

Pharmacists and doctors' offices throughout the United States and Europe sold and distributed cannabis throughout the second half of the 19th century to treat stomach problems and nausea, among other ailments. It was described in the *United States Pharmacopoeia* for the first time in 1851.[10,11]

Though it was widely used in the Middle East and parts of Asia for thousands of years, consuming marijuana to get high didn't catch on in the United States until the early 1900s, when, according to *Smoke Signals: A Social History of Marijuana—Medical, Recreational, and Scientific* by Martin A. Lee, immigrants from Mexico to the United States introduced the recreational practice of smoking marijuana to American culture.

When the Great Depression struck, public resentment of Mexican immigrants and, by association, marijuana grew. By 1931, 29 states had outlawed cannabis. In 1937, the Marijuana Tax Act was passed, imposing an inordinately high excise tax that effectively prohibited and punished the sale and use of cannabis. *The United States Pharmacopoeia* dropped cannabis from its pages in 1942.

The laws regarding possessing and using marijuana became increasingly stiff throughout the 1950s and early 1960s. President Richard Nixon signed the Controlled Substances Act of 1970, listing marijuana as a Schedule 1 substance (along with heroin and LSD), a category reserved for dangerous drugs with no medical use.

Public pressure would eventually result in a loosening of this policy. In 1996, California passed the Compassionate Use Act and became the first state to effectively legalize marijuana for medical use. Many other states would soon follow California's lead. As of late 2020, marijuana was legal for medical use in 38 states, though it is still illegal on the federal level.

our laws regarding cannabis and hemp have recently changed, opening the door for CBD production, sale, and consumption.

Botanically speaking, there are two broad categories of cannabis—industrial hemp plants and medicinal or drug plants. Industrial hemp plants tend to be tall, skinny, bamboo-like plants with skimpy foliage.

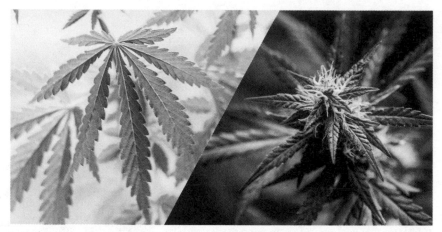

Industrial hemp plants (left) have skimpy foliage, while medicinal hemp plants (right) are bushy with lots of flowers.

These plants are machine harvested and manufactured into many different products like paper, cloth, and edible seed oil. Drug plants, by comparison, are bushy plants with lots of flowers, which is where most of the resin and the cannabinoids reside.

Until recently, U.S. federal law defined marijuana in terms of resin content. In 1970, the Controlled Substance Act (CSA) (which followed up on the 1937 Marijuana Tax Act before it) made certain parts of the cannabis plant, like the stalk and seed, exempt from the legal definition of "marihuana." But the flowers, the leaves, and the sticky resin and its derivatives were defined as marijuana and explicitly forbidden, even if the resin was only present in trace amounts.[12] Under these laws, CBD was illegal along with THC because it came from the resinous flowers, a forbidden part of the cannabis plant.

Things started to change when Congress passed the Agricultural Act of 2014 (otherwise known as the "Farm Bill"). Now, instead of any plant parts with sticky resin being lumped into the illegal "drug" category, cannabis could be considered "industrial hemp"[13]—*not marijuana*—as long as no part of the plant (including the leaves and flowers) exceeded a THC concentration of "more than 0.3 percent on a dry weight basis."

Though the 2014 Farm Bill relaxed the federal laws regarding hemp, its production was still subject to strict Drug Enforcement Administration (DEA) oversight, and only farmers associated with "institutes of higher education" and state agriculture departments could legally grow it with state government permission.

> Any plant topping 0.3 percent THC is considered marijuana and is federally illegal to grow.

Four years later, the laws loosened further. When the Agricultural Act or Farm Bill came due to be renewed in 2018, the bill was amended to legalize the production of hemp as an agricultural commodity and removed it from the list of controlled substances and DEA oversight. So now farmers could grow and produce cannabis, aka hemp, so long as it remains beneath that 0.3 percent THC threshold. Any plant that tops 0.3 percent THC is considered marijuana and is federally illegal to grow, though it is legal in the states that have approved the use of cannabis for therapeutic or adult recreational use (see "The State of Legal Cannabis," page 16).

If that sounds confusing, that's because it *is* confusing—to nearly everyone. This has been a good news, bad news situation for CBD and cannabis. On one hand, the Farm Bill *does* make it legal for American farmers to cultivate hemp as a commercial crop on domestic soil, and they are now growing it to feed the huge public demand for CBD.

On the other hand, advocates of the federal legalization of marijuana criticize the 0.3 percent THC legal limit as arbitrary and impractical. That 0.3 percent THC figure came from a 1976 journal article titled *A Practical and Natural Taxonomy of Cannabis*, which was designed to characterize cannabis varieties from a botanical perspective. It was never meant to be used as a legal doctrine, and cannabis advocates argue that using it as such impedes medical research and blocks access to valuable therapeutic options, including herbal extracts with various combinations of CBD and THC.[14]

It also creates a lot of confusion within the burgeoning CBD market. Legally speaking, hemp-derived CBD that contains less than the 0.3 percent THC cutoff is not considered a controlled substance. However, CBD oil derived from any cannabis plant with over 0.3 percent THC remains an illegal Schedule 1 substance under federal law. (Also, as of mid-2020, the FDA still maintains that hemp-derived CBD is neither a legitimate food supplement nor a medication approved for off-label use. That is likely to change at some point as the FDA relaxes its regulatory language; but at this time, it's further muddying the waters. More on that later.)

Contradictions within federal law and conflicts between state and federal law need to be reconciled in order to maximize the therapeutic potential of CBD. The ever-changing CBD landscape is bound to continue to grow and evolve as we continue to discover the myriad health benefits of this cannabis-based medicine.

CHAPTER

2

How CBD Works
in Your Body

T HE MORE SCIENTISTS study CBD, the more ways they find that it works to keep us healthy and happy. The latest research shows that CBD is a potent antioxidant, fights inflammation, promotes healthy metabolism, builds neurons, and protects the brain.

That's a lot of work for one molecule. But as you'll soon see, CBD doesn't do all these jobs by itself. Rather, it works with and within the cells of your body to optimize their performance. In other words, it helps you heal yourself and stay healthy. Here's how.

CBD and the Endocannabinoid System

One of CBD's chief roles is mimicking and augmenting the effects of our own natural cannabinoids, which are part of our endocannabinoid system.

That's right, humans make their own cannabinoids as part of what is called our endocannabinoid system, or ECS for short. The ECS plays a major role in brain function, immune activity, and maintaining equilibrium in our organ systems. Amazingly, scientists didn't even discover the endocannabinoid system until the 1990s!

Researchers discovered plant cannabinoids in the 1930s. Roger Adams, a chemist at the University of Illinois, was the first to identify and synthesize CBD in 1940. Picking up where Adams left off, Israeli scientist Raphael Mechoulam determined its molecular structure in 1963. As recreational cannabis use became widespread in the 1960s and 1970s, research expanded as scientists wanted to learn more about how cannabis altered our brain activity.[15]

Some researchers speculated that the human body may have receptors for these molecules, but it wasn't until the late 1980s that scientists identified them. As researchers dug deeper, they discovered that humans produced their own natural cannabinoids, and by the late 1990s researchers had mapped out the basics of the endocannabinoid system as we know it today. This discovery has significantly advanced our understanding of human biology, health, and disease.

It sounds almost outlandish, but since uncovering the inner workings of our innate endocannabinoid system, researchers have discovered that the ECS is dysregulated—meaning that it's impaired or otherwise not functioning normally—in nearly *all* disease states, including cancer, diabetes, Alzheimer's, chronic pain, sleep disorders, and addiction, just to name a few.

The health benefits of balancing the ECS are so profound that in 2013, U.S. National Institutes of Health (NIH) scientists Pal Pacher and George Kunos declared that "modulating endocannabinoid system activity may have therapeutic potential in almost all diseases affecting humans."[16]

Since CBD can modulate the endocannabinoid system, it's easy to see how this molecule has gotten so much attention lately.

The Endocannabinoid System: The Master Regulator

Italian scientist Vincenzo DiMarzo described the role of the endocannabinoid system in human health as helping us to "eat, sleep, relax, protect, and forget."[17] Let's take a closer look at these five key functions:

You Name It, the ECS Regulates It

It's natural to be skeptical that one product could possibly protect against and provide relief from the wide array of conditions people use CBD for. But when you look at the long list of biological functions that your endocannabinoid system regulates, it makes perfect sense! This is just a partial list of functions your ECS manages:

- Appetite & digestion
- Blood pressure
- Bone density & growth
- Cardiovascular function
- Energy metabolism
- Fertility

- Fibrosis
- Inflammation
- Liver function
- Memory
- Mood
- Muscle formation

- Neuroprotection & neurogenesis
- Pain
- Sexual function
- Skin & nerve function
- Sleep
- Stress[18]

Eat: The ECS helps regulate appetite and satiety.

Sleep: It helps you wind down and get a good night's sleep.

Relax: The ECS promotes physical and mental well-being by mitigating stress.

Protect: It builds brain cells to protect your brain health, promotes healthy metabolism, and modulates your immune system so that it can fend off harmful invaders.

Forget: Seems like an odd one here, but forgetting is an essential component of healthy living. If you remembered every single detail of what happened every second of every day, you wouldn't be able to function like a sane person. The ECS regulates both essential memory and "memory extinction," forgetting what's not important to remember.

How does the ECS do all these things? By acting as a master regulator for your body. Imagine you're sitting in a room surrounded by four walls covered with 100 thermostats. Each of these thermostats regulates an essential physiological function that keeps us safe and

Distribution of Cannabinoid Receptors in Brain

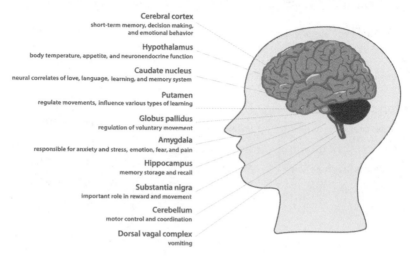

Cerebral cortex
short-term memory, decision making,
and emotional behavior

Hypothalamus
body temperature, appetite, and neuronendocrine function

Caudate nucleus
neural correlates of love, language, learning, and memory system

Putamen
regulate movements, influence various types of learning

Globus pallidus
regulation of voluntary movement

Amygdala
responsible for anxiety and stress, emotion, fear, and pain

Hippocampus
memory storage and recall

Substantia nigra
important role in reward and movement

Cerebellum
motor control and coordination

Dorsal vagal complex
vomiting

Cannabinoid receptors are found throughout the brain, where they can influence many different systems throughout the body.

comfortable. Think of the ECS as the sum total of all those thermostats combined into a single, dynamic system that's involved in regulating nearly all human biological activity.

As the master regulator, the ECS controls a broad array of physiological processes like wound healing, blood pressure, pain perception, brain cell production, glucose metabolism, and immune function to control inflammation. When you're faced with an emergency situation, you get a surge of stress hormones like cortisol and adrenaline so you can act appropriately—"fight or flight," as it's commonly known. Once the threat is no longer present and the situation returns to normal, your ECS turns down the stress response and brings those hormones back to baseline.

Likewise, when you're sick and you need a fever to fight and kill whatever bug you have, the ECS turns up the heat.[19] And when the invader is eliminated and you no longer need the fever, the ECS turns down the immune system's dimmer switch to bring your temperature back to normal. Autoimmune diseases are an expression of ECS dysfunction. When that ECS dimmer switch is broken, your body can't turn down the inflammatory response, and your healthy tissues become damaged. As mentioned earlier (and you'll learn in detail in the next section), many diseases are an expression of a poorly functioning or dysfunctional ECS.

The Inner Workings of the Endocannabinoid System

Researchers continue to study the intricacies of the inner workings of the endocannabinoid system, so our understanding continues to evolve. But the basics are well established.

These are the three chief components to the ECS that were discovered by scientists in the 1990s:

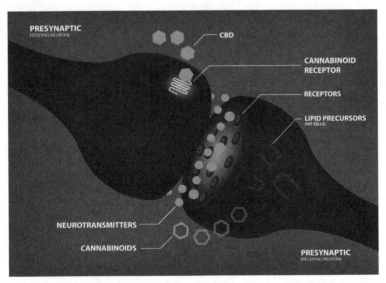

When a cannabinoid binds to a cannabinoid receptor, it sets off chemical reactions that can affect behavior, mood, and more.

Cannabinoid receptors: These are like miniature portals that sit on the surface of cells throughout our brain, central nervous system, and other organs. They pick up important signals about what's going on in the body so those cells can take appropriate actions as needed. There are two main types of cannabinoid receptors: CB_1 and CB_2. Both are scattered throughout your body, but CB_1 receptors are concentrated in your brain and central nervous system and CB_2 receptors are concentrated in your immune system. Both types of cannabinoid receptors are present in the skin, liver, kidneys, heart, and other internal organs.

Endocannabinoids: These are molecules that attach to cannabinoid receptors and activate them like a key turning a lock. Scientists have discovered more than a dozen endocannabinoids within our bodies, but two are most prevalent: *2-Arachidonoylglycerol (2AG)* and *anandamide*, named for the Sanskrit word *ananda*, meaning bliss, because of its reputation as a mood enhancer. These interact with the same receptors as THC and other components of the cannabis plant.

"I Tried It"

Stephanie Johnson, 47,
Dallas, Texas

Stephanie Johnson was diagnosed with advanced, triple-negative breast cancer when she was 38. "I was given a 23 percent chance of living to see five years, and now I'm at eight years," says Johnson. "I got to see my boys become men." Her sons, teens at the time, are now 22 and 25.

After her diagnosis, Johnson endured a year of treatment that included four months of chemotherapy and three surgeries. But while the chemo drug, Taxol, helped eliminate her cancer, it left Johnson with painful nerve damage in her hands and feet that she continues to struggle with today. Johnson likens the sensation to being stabbed with a multitude of tiny icepicks. "It's prickly and almost an electrical shock feeling. The feet will swell and get sore, too."

Her condition, peripheral neuropathy, can also result from poorly con-

Metabolic enzymes: These enzymes are proteins that accelerate chemical reactions. They are involved in both creating endocannabinoids when needed and breaking them down and destroying them once the endocannabinoids have served their purpose.

CBD, a Molecular VIP

More recently, a fourth component of the ECS was discovered—the transport molecules that act like shuttles for endocannabinoids, ferrying them to where they need to go. Known as fatty acid binding proteins, these transports are also key to how CBD does its job.

When scientists first discovered our natural *endogenous* cannabinoids (2AG and anandamide, the ones we create ourselves),[21] they wondered how they made their way through the body's aqueous interior. After all, blood is mainly water and cannabinoids are fatty lipids—and oil and water are famous for not mixing very well. The key breakthrough came in 2009 with the identification of specific transport molecules for endogenous cannabinoids.

As the name indicates, those fatty acid binding proteins attach

trolled diabetes, autoimmune disease, nutritional deficiency, viral infections, and many other factors. For about 18 months, Johnson tried treating her tingling hands and feet with over-the-counter pain relievers and topicals. But she couldn't find relief—plus, she worried about potential side effects, like organ damage. "I finally was like, you know what, I'll try this CBD stuff," she says. Johnson had become familiar with CBD through her job at a marketing, branding, and advertising agency in Dallas, where she researched and wrote content for clients, including CBD product makers, hemp farmers, and medical marijuana firms.

Johnson felt the effects of CBD right away. "I remember the first time I tried a topical on my feet," she said. "I could feel the pain calming down and everything subsiding, and I looked at my husband and said, 'I feel good! This is great!'" She has tried an array of CBD products before settling on a cream she uses anytime the pain flares up, plus a CBD oil to ease achy legs at bedtime.[20]

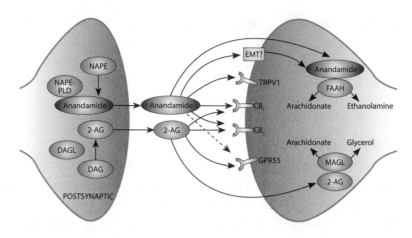

Endocannabinoids form within neurons and then cross the synaptic cleft between cells.

to fatty lipids like cannabinoids. In your bloodstream, these fatty acid binding proteins function like a molecular canoe that picks up cannabinoids and shuttles them to where they need to go, including through the cell membrane and inside the cell, where they interact with receptors on the surface of the cell's nucleus.[22] Known as *peroxisome proliferator-activated receptors*, or *PPARs*, these nuclear receptors regulate gene expression and energy metabolism, as well as other important physiological processes. CBD, it turns out, is a VIP passenger on those same canoes, and this may have a lot to do with why CBD can have such profound therapeutic effects.

When you take CBD, it's as if it elbows its way to the front of the cannabinoid line, pushes aside 2AG and anandamide, and takes priority seating on the canoe. That means that your natural cannabinoids hang around on the surface of your cells longer, which gives them more time to activate your CB_1 and CB_2 receptors, until the next ride comes along to transport your endocannabinoids inside the cell, where they are ultimately deactivated by metabolic enzymes.

In essence, CBD acts a "reuptake inhibitor" that prolongs the natural life cycle of our own natural endocannabinoids so they can confer more therapeutic benefits. Much like you tone weak biceps by lifting weights and exposing your muscle fibers to extra muscle-making stimulus, CBD boosts the "tone" of your endocannabinoid system by exposing it to an extended dose of cannabinoid activity. Scientists believe this may be a key mechanism whereby CBD helps to protect the brain, buffer stress, and fight disease.

> CBD helps to protect the brain, buffer stress, and fight disease.

CBD, Cellular Volume Control

Hogging space on those canoes and extending the lifespan of 2AG and anandamide is one way that CBD helps to improve endocannabinoid tone. But that's not the only way CBD interacts with your endocannabinoid system. In addition to increasing the levels of endocannabinoids by delaying their reuptake and metabolic breakdown, CBD can also alter and adjust how your cannabinoid receptors function.

THC binds directly to both CB_1 and CB_2 cannabinoid receptors like a key fitting into a lock and activates these receptors, causing them to send a signal that culminates in a physiological response (less pain, less inflammation, lower blood pressure, relaxation, etc.). But CBD doesn't work this way. Instead of binding with cannabinoid receptors to initiate a signal itself, CBD fine-tunes the signaling that's been triggered by THC or an endogenous cannabinoid.

Researchers are still trying to figure out exactly how CBD does this, and the science is very much a work in progress, but here's a glimpse of what we know thus far. Preclinical (in vitro) studies indicate that CBD functions as an *allosteric modulator* at the CB_1 receptor, meaning that it influences how the receptor signals without actually causing it to signal. Think of the CB_1 receptor as a dimmer switch or volume control knob—CBD turns it down slightly but not all the way. This appears to be one of the mechanisms whereby CBD lowers the ceiling on THC's tricky psychoactivity and lessens the high, which is caused by direct CB_1 receptor activation.

At the same time, CBD augments CB_2 receptor signaling, which regulates inflammation and immune cell activity. How and why CBD triggers an anti-inflammatory response and other CB_2-mediated outcomes without directly binding to the CB_2 receptor is still somewhat of a scientific mystery. But this much is evident: CBD can fine-tune the ECS by modulating CB_1 and CB_2 receptor activity in different directions, tempering the former while amplifying the latter. And this combination can have profound, health-positive effects, particularly for metabolic disorders, obesity, liver disease, and other diseases linked to the Western diet (see page 47).

To recap: CBD can elevate the levels of your endogenous cannabinoid compounds, anandamide and 2AG, which activate your cannabinoid receptors and cause them to signal. CBD can also fine-tune the way your cannabinoid receptors function, turning down the volume at CB_1 while augmenting CB_2 in a manner that balances the body and promotes good health.

3

The Swiss Army Knife of Natural Healing

C BD'S INFLUENCE ON the endocannabinoid system is a key way in which the molecule helps to prevent disease and improve health and well-being, but it's not the only way it works.

Extensive preclinical research (the kind done in labs and on animals before human studies can be conducted) suggests that CBD has a lot of "anti" powers. Specifically, it's anti-tumoral, inhibiting tumor development; anti-spasmodic, suppressing muscle spasms; anti-convulsive, preventing seizures; and anxiolytic, inhibiting anxiety. It's also neuroprotective, so it helps promote brain health.[23]

Some of these benefits are related to how CBD reacts with the ECS, but not all of them trace back to that system. Understanding how CBD exerts its myriad effects on human physiology is a work in progress. So far, scientists have identified more than 65 different molecular pathways through which CBD operates.[24] The more researchers learn about this versatile molecule, the more they appreciate that it's like a Swiss army knife of therapeutic benefits.

For example, CBD interacts with a number of other kinds of receptors (aside from the CB receptors), on your cells' membranes. And when it hitches a ride on our canoe (the fatty acid binding protein), CBD is transported through the cell membrane into the watery interior of the cell, where the phytocannabinoid interacts with more receptors, providing additional protection and benefits, including:

Fighting Free Radicals (Especially in the Brain)

CBD and other cannabinoids mitigate free-radical damage by acting as extremely potent antioxidants, and this offers a huge array of health benefits.

The human body is under constant oxidative stress. When your cells use oxygen to create energy, they produce waste products called *free radicals*—atoms with an odd number of electrons that steal electrons from other atoms in a tissue-damaging game of molecular musical chairs.

"I Tried It"

Michelle Smith, 57
St. Augustine, Florida

About two years ago, Michelle Smith noticed she was having trouble falling and staying asleep. She started to wake up more during the night. She wanted something that would calm the racing thoughts that popped up as soon as her head hit the pillow. "It's hard for me to shut down at night," she says. "That's why [some] people turn to alcohol and things like that. I was trying to find something that would do that without all the [bad] side effects."

After both a friend and her massage therapist recommended CBD for her anxiety, she decided to give it a try. "Now when I go to bed, I'm able to let go of what's happened during the day and not worry about what's coming up tomorrow," says Smith. "I felt relaxed the first time I took it, but it's not a magic pill. There's nothing about it that feels like a high. It feels like I just took a deep breath."

Smith says her anxiety kicked into high gear as an adult after her son was diagnosed with an

Your body has its own natural free-radical fighters called *antioxidants*, which offer their own electrons to stop the marauding molecules in their tracks before they can do their damage.

Sometimes there are more free radicals than antioxidants to neutralize them, and your body's natural defenses get overwhelmed. When that happens, free radicals can go so far as to steal from your DNA, which can lead to myriad diseases including heart disease, cancer, and stroke. This process is called *oxidation*, and it's what makes a sliced apple turn brown when exposed to the air. When you squeeze lemon juice on apple slices, you're giving them antioxidant protection. When you eat vitamin C–rich citrus fruit, you're giving yourself that same antioxidant protection.

That's why it's important to eat a healthy diet rich in fruits and vegetables that deliver extra antioxidants to fortify your natural free-radical fighting system. Vitamins C, E, and beta-carotene are well-known antioxidants.

autoimmune disease and required two liver transplants during his childhood. The intense caregiving combined with the stress of the breakup of her marriage led to an anxiety disorder diagnosis. She was prescribed sertraline (Zoloft)—a medication that can help regulate mood. Then she went to counseling. But over the years, she began taking a more holistic approach to her mental and physical health. She was able to stop taking Zoloft, and her regimen now includes eating mostly vegetarian, daily meditation, exercising at least five days a week, and CBD. Each night about half an hour before bed, Smith takes half a dropperful of CBD tincture, which contains about 20 mg per dose.

These days, Smith's son is 22 and in good health. Adjusting to this new normal has been both a blessing and a challenge for her, after spending so many years primed to go into panic mode and never knowing when the next medical emergency would strike. "I've spent a lot of my time in fight-or-flight mode, and that is exhausting, so being able to calm down and rest my body and my mind is important. People think self-care is selfish, but it's not. It's necessary. And for me, CBD is part of that holistic approach."[25]

According to a 1998 study, CBD and THC are even more powerful antioxidants than vitamins C and E. Much like these vitamins, cannabinoids perform their antioxidant activity best when they work together with all the other natural chemicals in the cannabis plant to create an entourage effect. Cannabinoids' antioxidant powers seem particularly helpful for brain health.

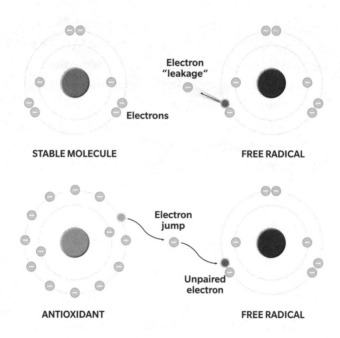

Antioxidants like CBD help protect your body and brain tissue from damage by free radicals.

In 2003, the U.S. Department of Health and Human Services received a patent on cannabinoids based on research into CBD and THC (such patents are intended to make sure that discoveries made by government scientists are utilized to benefit the public).[26] That patent was titled "Cannabinoids as antioxidants and neuroprotectants." In it, the department concluded:

Cannabinoids have been found to have antioxidant properties [and] are found to have particular application as neuroprotectants, for example in limiting neurological damage following ischemic insults, such as stroke and trauma, or in the treatment of neuro-degenerative diseases, such as Alzheimer's disease, Parkinson's disease and HIV dementia.

Quelling Inflammation

Inflammation in small doses is a good thing. It's how your body mounts defenses against injury and infection, like how you get a fever when you have the flu and swelling from a twisted ankle. But *systemic inflammation*, which is a low-level inflammation you don't readily see or feel, can happen even when there's no real illness or injury to fight and is the root cause of many chronic diseases.

There are many culprits that cause systemic inflammation:
- too much stress;
- lack of quality sleep;
- being overweight (especially if you carry your excess fat in your abdomen, where it is most metabolically active);
- a diet high in processed foods, like sodas, chips, hot dogs, and sugary breakfast cereals;
- exposure to secondhand smoke and other pollutants.

The result is that your body starts fighting itself, damaging healthy organs, tissues, blood vessels, and joints. Left unchecked, systemic inflammation can lead to many serious diseases like heart disease, diabetes, stroke, arthritis, irritable bowel disease, neurodegenerative diseases like Alzheimer's, and some cancers.

A review study published in *Future Medicinal Chemistry* found that phytocannabinoids like CBD suppress the inflammatory response and can be an effective treatment for reducing systemic inflammation.[27] Being a powerful antioxidant also makes CBD good at fighting inflammation. A 2011 study published in *Free Radical Biology and Medicine* concluded that CBD showed potential for lowering inflammation related to free radical stress that occurs when rogue molecules steal electrons from your healthy cells, damaging DNA and triggering the body's inflammatory immune response. [28, 29]

Animal research published in 2020 by James M. Nichols and Barbara L.F. Kaplan of Mississippi State University reported that CBD's anti-inflammatory action provides a host of important health benefits, including reducing inflammation in the brain and lungs.[30] In people with epilepsy, it also reduces seizure severity, frequency, and recovery time. This is key, because seizure activity induces brain inflammation, which can become chronic with repeated seizures.[31]

CBD's anti-inflammatory properties augment the activity of your CB_2 receptors, which are concentrated on your immune cells—your body's front line defense against pathogens that trigger inflammation.[32] CBD and the CB_2 receptor both reduce the inflammatory immune response. Suppressing immune function might not sound like an obvious benefit, but in the case of autoimmune diseases, which affect nearly 25 million Americans in the form of multiple sclerosis, rheumatoid arthritis, irritable bowel disease, lupus, and others, the immune system promotes disease rather than protecting against it. In these cases, immune system suppression has a protective, healing benefit.[33]

Turning On and Off Genes

There's a saying in genetic circles that your genes load the gun and the environment pulls the trigger. So you may have genes that predispose you to certain diseases or conditions, but unless you do something that turns them on or off, you may never actually get those diseases or conditions.

CBD is emerging as a key player for influencing gene expression. For instance, CBD silences a gene known as ID-1, which, when activated, is linked to the metastatic process that spreads cancer cells from the original tumor throughout the body. In fact, the ID-1 gene is found only in metastatic cancer cells. By "silencing" or deactivating this gene, CBD may help in treating certain aggressive forms of cancer without the troubling and painful side effects of chemotherapy.

In 2012, Israeli scientists identified more than 1,200 genes that are either turned on or off by cannabidiol in an experiment that focused on CBD's role in zinc homeostasis, which has a direct bearing on immune function. In the same experiment, THC was found to regulate 94 genes. "The results show that CBD, but much less so THC, affects the expression of genes involved in zinc homeostasis and suggest that the regulation of zinc levels could have an important role through which CBD may exert its antioxidant and anti-inflammatory effects," the Israeli research team concluded.[34]

> CBD may help treat cancer without painful side effects.

One of the ways CBD influences the expression of genes is by binding to what are known as PPARs, which sit on the surface of the cell's nucleus. These receptors are instrumental in regulating energy balance and gene expression. Laboratory research shows that activating a PPAR receptor known as *PPAR-gamma* can prevent cancer cell proliferation and even make tumors shrink in studies on human lung cancer cells.

CBD is a PPAR-gamma "agonist," which means that it activates this receptor. Activating PPAR-gamma receptors also facilitates the breakdown of amyloid-beta plaque, a key molecule linked to the development of Alzheimer's disease. This is one of the reasons why CBD may be a useful supplement for Alzheimer's patients. PPAR receptors are also involved in regulating insulin sensitivity, which helps to explain why CBD is useful for preventing and treating diabetes, according to animal studies and anecdotal accounts from CBD consumers.

Building Brain Cells

One broad effect of both CBD and THC is the stimulation of neurogenesis—the production and integration of new neurons in the brain. Research shows that CBD increases the production of *brain-derived neurotrophic factor* (BDNF), a naturally occurring protein that acts like Miracle-Gro for your brain. BDNF encourages the growth of new neurons and improves the health of existing brain cells. BDNF also helps build and maintain connections between neurons.

Exercise has been shown to pump up the production of BDNF. So does CBD. This, along with CBD's antioxidant and anti-inflammatory properties, makes CBD a powerful neuroprotectant, meaning it's really good for brain health.

Regulating Blood Pressure, Bone Density, and Cell Growth

CBD binds with a number of orphan receptors, which bear that name because scientists aren't sure which endogenous compounds (those your body produces naturally) activate or block these receptors. One such orphan receptor is GPR55.

GPR55 is involved in regulating blood pressure. By binding to it, CBD can promote vasodilation (the widening of blood vessels) and lower blood pressure.[35] It is also responsible for facilitating bone reabsorption, where the body breaks down your bones. This is part of the natural bone-remodeling process that allows your skeleton to regenerate over time and release minerals. Scientists have found that overactive GPR55 receptor signaling is linked to osteoporosis. CBD is a GPR55 antagonist, meaning that it blocks this receptor from signaling. Research suggests that by blocking GPR55 signaling, CBD acts to decrease bone reabsorption. If unchecked, bone reabsorption can accelerate over time, leading to poor remodeling and bone thinning.[36] By mitigating bone reabsorption, CBD prevents osteoporosis.

A similar mechanism involving GPR55 may also help to fight cancer.

A 2010 study by researchers at the Chinese Academy of Scientists reported that GPR55 activation promotes the aggressive proliferation of cancer cells.[37] By blocking GPR55 from signaling, CBD could help stop the rapid reproduction of cancer cells.

Managing Mood and Pain Perception

CBD also binds to a receptor known as TRPV1, which plays an important role in pain perception, inflammation, and body temperature. This receptor is part of a large family of so-called "trip" receptors, which regulate visceral sensations such as heat and cold, light sensitivity, and pain. Various herbs and spices (such as mustard, peppermint, and peppers) activate these receptors. Capsaicin—the pungent compound in hot chile peppers also commonly used for pain relief—activates the TRPV1 receptor. So does CBD and our endogenous "bliss molecule," anandamide.

In addition, CBD binds to several serotonin receptor subtypes. Serotonin is an important chemical messenger that helps regulate your moods, appetite, digestion, sleep, memory, pain perception, and more. It has been called the "happy chemical" because it contributes to feelings of well-being. Research shows that high concentrations of CBD directly activate a serotonin receptor known as hydroxytryptamine (5-HT1A), which helps ease anxiety. It may also help to improve sleep, prevent nausea, and fight addiction and appetite disorders.

Gamma-aminobutyric acid (GABA) is another chemical messenger that is widely distributed in your brain. GABA inhibits chemical messengers in your nervous system. It's like volume control for the brain, turning down the noise so you're more relaxed. Powerful pharmaceutical drugs like Valium, Xanax, and other benzodiazepines turn the volume *way* down by binding to GABA receptors. CBD works in a different way, making it easier for GABA receptors to bind with the body's own GABA molecules, thereby enhancing their natural calming effect.

An Interview with a Neuroscientist

Greg Gerdeman, PhD

The discovery of the endocannabinoid system has major implications for nearly every area of medical science and helps to explain how and why CBD and THC are such versatile therapeutic compounds. Martin A. Lee of Project CBD interviewed Greg Gerdeman, PhD, a neuroscientist who specializes in cannabinoid research. This edited conversation answers basic questions many people have about the endocannabinoid system.[38]

Project CBD: *What does the endo-cannabinoid system mean in terms of neuroscience?*

Gerdeman: The cannabinoid receptors and the endocannabinoids that act on them are abundant throughout the nervous system. The brain, the spinal cord, and the peripheral nerves maintain a state of safe operation by using endocannabinoids and similar molecules. Plus, we now know that everything from Alzheimer's to motor disorders to head trauma are related to neural inflammation. Both endo-cannabinoids and plant cannabinoids dampen that down, so the therapeutic potential is tremendous.

Project CBD: *What about neural plasticity—the brain's ability to remodel itself in response to injury? What role does the endocannabinoid system play in that?*

Gerdeman: Endocannabinoids are involved in how the connections between brain cell—called synapses—rearrange and rewire themselves. Synaptic or neural plasticity is how learning and memory of all kinds works. Certain things like exercise and living in a social environment promote neurogenesis (the promotion of new brain cells). It's believed that this helps to improve emotional well-being. The endocannabinoid system is very much involved in that. We know it because, if animals don't have cannabinoid receptors or if they are blocked by drugs, they do not experience the same level of neurogenesis.

With head injury, stroke, with other kinds of chronic trauma that leads to inflammation and cell death, neural plasticity and the generation of new neurons is part of rehabilitation. CBD can help to stimulate and support that neurogenesis. For example, I have witnessed people begin taking good-quality CBD oil right after they've had a head injury, only to recover far better than their neurologist expected.

mechanism by which cells communicate with their neighbors and help to keep the whole body function. Discovering the endocannabinoid system has advanced our understanding of the biology of being well. It has taught us how exercise works and how we are truly meant to be active, dynamic beings, and that's part of health. And that inflammation is so critical to chronic illness—all these doors have been opened by studying the endocannabinoid system and how it responds to plant cannabinoids.

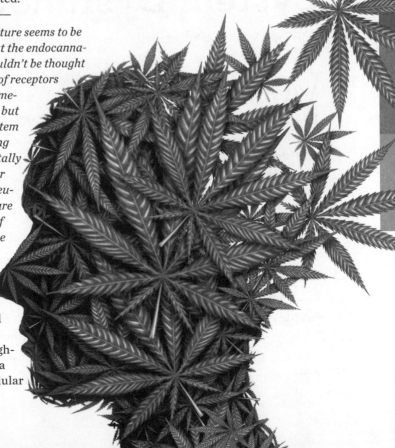

Project CBD: *A picture seems to be emerging such that the endocannabinoid system shouldn't be thought of just as a bunch of receptors that respond to something in cannabis, but as an amazing system that's really helping us stay fundamentally healthy. From your perspective as a neuroscientist, what are the implications of the discovery of the endocannabinoid system?*

Gerdeman: The endocannabinoid system is fully integrated throughout the body. It's a fundamental cellular

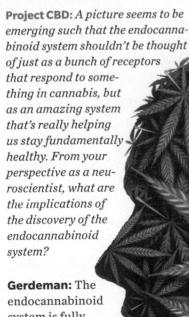

4

What Causes Endocannabinoid System Dysfunction?

WHEN YOUR ENDOCANNABINOID system is running on all cylinders, it can perform its duty well as your master regulator, keeping your hormones, immunity, and metabolism humming along in homeostasis.

Unfortunately, the endocannabinoid system is not immune to dysfunction, deficiency, and overreaction. In some cases, it appears that the body simply doesn't produce enough endocannabinoids or enough receptors that function properly for the endocannabinoid system to perform the way it should—which opens the door for disease.

In 2004, neurologist Ethan Russo, MD, a prominent cannabinoid researcher, introduced the concept of "clinical endocannabinoid deficiency."[39] He proposed that diminished endocannabinoid function is at the root of several pathologies. Initially, Russo mentioned three diseases—migraines, fibromyalgia, and irritable bowel syndrome (IBS, also known as spastic colon)—which often appear as a cluster of symptoms in patients who are cannabinoid deficient.

Subsequent studies by other scientists would lend credence to Russo's thesis by linking endocannabinoid deficits to various aberrant conditions, including epilepsy, PTSD, autism, alcoholism, clinical depression, and other neurodegenerative ailments.

Thankfully, there are things we can do to tone our endocannabinoid system so it works better. It makes sense that CBD and other holistic healing techniques that enhance cannabinoid receptor signaling may be viable treatment strategies for endocannabinoid deficiency disorders.

Our Stressed-Out Endocannabinoid System

Chronic stress is one of the biggest drains on our endocannabinoid system, and a huge portion of the population suffers from it. We have demanding jobs and hectic home lives, and we are bombarded with bad news from around the world at every turn. According to an April 2020 Gallup Poll, Americans' stress levels have risen during the COVID-19 pandemic with 60 percent of adults reporting that they felt significant stress the day before, a full 14 points higher than is typical.[40] A 2019 *Consumer Reports* survey of more than 4,000 Americans found that 37 percent of those who use CBD listed stress reduction as the number-one reason they use it.[41]

There is more than one type of stress, and it's not all bad. You need acute stress to survive. When faced with a dangerous situation, your emergency "fight-or-flight" system (scientifically known as your hypothalamic-pituitary-adrenal, or HPA, axis) fires up and creates an influx of stress hormones like adrenaline and cortisol, which gives you the burst of energy you need to do what you have to do to survive. Once the danger has passed, your endocannabinoid system (ECS) kicks in to increase levels of endocannabinoids to help bring your body down from high alert and back to pre-stress levels.

Chronic stress is different. When you're exposed to even low levels of constant stress, your ECS becomes worn out. Now, instead of your

The Runner's High:
It's Not about the Endorphins

Exercise enthusiasts have extolled the wonders of the "runner's high" for decades. Endorphins, related to the body's opiate system, have long gotten the credit for that euphoric feeling following, and sometimes during, a long, hard workout. But now scientists know that state of exercise bliss is also a product of endocannabinoids.[42]

"When you get to a certain level of real elation or a zone that feels kind of out-of-body that can be due to opiates like endorphins," says Greg Gerdeman, PhD, a neuroscientist who studies cannabis and the endocannabinoid system.[43] "But there is an endocannabinoid-mediated 'runner's joy' or a 'runner's bliss,' if you will, to play with the name of anandamide (meaning bliss)."

In a study, Gerdeman and his colleagues monitored runners for 30 minutes reaching an aerobic training zone of 50 to 70 percent of their max heart rate. As they were running, their anandamide levels rose, as did their mood, leaving them in a "joy state."[44]

The phenomenon is likely grounded in our roots as hunters and gatherers, Gerdeman says.

"Human beings evolved to be movers, to be exercisers, to be endurance runners. What motivated our hominid ancestors to start running long distances? Part of that answer is the endocannabinoid system being utilized by the brain to feel good and also to regulate your energy," he says. "The endocannabinoids help to improve how much you enjoy food, which is the object of our running, foraging behavior, evolutionarily speaking."

ECS bringing you back to baseline, it takes a downturn. Chronic stress depletes endocannabinoid tone. It not only blunts CB_1 activity, but also increases levels of *fatty acid amide hydrolase* (FAAH), the enzyme that breaks anandamide down in the body, resulting in lower concentrations of the feel-good endocannabinoid.

With weakened endocannabinoid signaling, we are more vulnerable to developing anxiety and depression. Indeed, one study showed a clear inverse relationship between anandamide levels and anxiety severity in women with major depression.[45] So, in basic terms, the more endocannabinoid deficient we are, the more anxious we tend to become.

Chronic stress and poor ECS tone also leave us with elevated levels of the stress hormone cortisol. Two-thirds of people with depression have high cortisol levels. Excess cortisol also contributes to systemic inflammation, weight gain, hypertension, high blood sugar, impaired immune function, hormone imbalances, cognitive impairment, and the likelihood of developing an autoimmune disorder.

Many of us also live in a highly polluted environment. More than 40 percent of Americans live with unhealthy air day in and day out. The same percentage of Americans say they don't get enough sleep. All of this contributes to our chronic stress load and to endocannabinoid deficiency.

Diet, Exercise, and Endocannabinoid Tone

When it is working properly, the endocannabinoid system keeps our appetite, satiety, and weight finely balanced. CB_1 receptors in our brain are responsible for signaling that it's time to eat when we need food, rousing our appetite and sharpening our sense of smell so food is extra rewarding. CB_2 receptor activation, on the other hand, works to reduce food intake and prevent the buildup of body fat.

Back in ancient times, when only fresh meat, fruits, and vegetables were available to eat, it was easier to naturally keep our ECS in balance. But our diet is so out of whack in the modern world that our CB_1 receptors are stuck in overdrive mode, reinforcing an aberrant feed-reward-feed loop from all the sugary, high-fat foods we consume. One study on mice found that when the rodents were fed a diet high in fat and sugar for 60 days, their CB_1 receptors became overactive, which prevented the secretion of amino acids meant to reduce appetite when the system is working properly. On the other hand, our CB_2 receptors—which are activated by plant-based foods like leafy and bitter greens, olive oil, and various spices—are essentially undernourished in a typical Western diet that's heavy on carbs and processed food.[46]

Omega-3 fatty acid deficiencies also distort how our cannabinoid receptors function. These healthful fatty acids keep our ECS humming along smoothly. But when you are deficient in omega-3 fatty acids (as many Americans are), your ECS function becomes impaired.

The health of your gut microbiome (the trillions of bacteria that live in your gut) is also essential and not just because it aids with effective and efficient digestion.[47] Your gut has a "brain" of its own that communicates with the brain between your ears. Medical scientists recognize the importance of the gut-brain axis, which influences inflammation, digestion, and even your moods, emotions, and general well-being. The ECS regulates your gut-brain axis, facilitating communication between the microbiome and the brain. If your diet is damaging your microbiome and causing gut dysbiosis, it's also skewing your ECS and the way your brain functions.

Physical activity (like we used to do to hunt, grow, and gather our food) is also essential to maintain good endocannabinoid tone. Exercise triggers the release of your natural endocannabinoids, helping you maintain lower stress levels and a healthy weight.[48] But it's all too easy these days to spend most of our time sitting—in front of our desks, in the car, or on the couch.

The cumulative result of poor lifestyle habits: ECS dysfunction and metabolic syndrome, heart disease, and other degenerative conditions associated with our heavily processed Western diet and sedentary lifestyle.

Rebalancing the Endocannabinoid System

Low ECS tone and the chronic inflammation and metabolic havoc that follow paves the way for many diseases. Studies published in a variety of medical journals have suggested that migraines, fibromyalgia, irritable bowel disease, depression, Alzheimer's, epilepsy, autism, and alcoholism all involve ECS dysregulation. Inflammation is also inextricably linked to pain and contributes to or speeds up the progression of many conditions from cancer to the common cold.

By boosting your natural cannabinoids, CBD enhances your ECS function and reduces stress and inflammation and their detrimental effects.[49] Medical scientists are hopeful—and research is starting to show—that this can help us treat and relieve a wide array of diseases, as we'll cover in more detail in Part II.

It's important to note here, however, that CBD can't completely make up for a poor diet, sedentary habits, and chronic stress. Taking CBD to improve your endocannabinoid tone will work best if you also pair it with lifestyle behaviors that support, rather than deplete, your ECS. If you take CBD during the day and subsist on chips and beer

---

"I Tried It"

Terrell Davis, 47
Los Angeles, California

As a professional football player, Terrell Davis' body has been through a lot of stress over the years. "Day-to-day pain management became my reality on the field and extended well into retirement," he said. So when Davis heard the praises of CBD from colleagues and trainers, it was a no-brainer that he give it a try. The results, he says, have been transformative to his life.

With a knee injury that often flares up as well as sore areas after workouts, Davis had been searching for the best form of relief. CBD was his solution. "To have a natural product that works as well if not better than harmful pills has been a boon to my success," Davis said. "At 47 years old, I am hitting the gym every day with the same vigor as my 20s."

Davis regularly uses a CBD oil from which 100 percent of the residual THC is eliminated. Since starting to use CBD, Davis has completely stopped using pain medication. "The need for NSAIDs and other OTC pain medication has nearly vanished," Davis said. "I can't even tell you the last time I have reached for pills, thanks to CBD."

In addition to taking CBD oil, Davis also smooths CBD balm over the affected area for fast pain relief. "If I'm suffering from a flare-up in my knee due to injury or a particularly sore area following a tough workout, I add in the CBD muscle balm with menthol and camphor, which feels amazing and gives me relief in minutes," Davis said.

while pulling an all-nighter, you're making it more difficult to benefit from CBD.

Regular exercise is crucial to boost endocannabinoid signaling (which is the mechanism behind that runner's high you get following a good workout). More research is needed to determine how much and what type of exercise is best for ECS tone. One study found that runners and cyclists exercising for 50 minutes experienced dramatic increases in anandamide, for instance.[50] A 2019 study published in *Medicine & Science in Sports & Exercise* reported that even 30 minutes of moderate-intensity exercise can boost endocannabinoid levels. Physical activity also helps you relieve stress and get a good night's sleep, which in turn help fortify the ECS.[51] Meditating, taking a relaxing bath, connecting with loved ones, and finding other healthy ways of coping with stress are also key. If you have sleep issues, CBD may be able to help (see page 121).

The foods that help boost endocannabinoid tone are the same ones you would find in traditionally healthful diets like the Mediterranean diet. Likewise, foods that support a healthy gut microbiome also improve ECS function. Minimize sugary, fatty, and overly processed foods. Instead, focus on getting more:

- **Fruits and vegetables** (especially those such as leeks, onions, asparagus, and garlic, which are known to improve gut health)

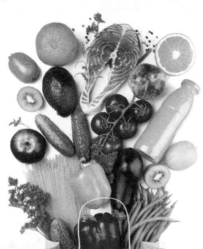

- **Foods that are good sources of omega-3 fatty acids**, including salmon and other fatty fish, walnuts, and flax and hemp seeds[52]
- **Fermented foods** such as yogurt, kefir, sauerkraut, and kimchi
- **Lean meat, eggs, and dairy products** are also sources of arachidonic acid, the chemical building block of endocannabinoids, but most Americans already get more than they need of these foods.

5

CBD Myths & Facts

C BD'S SKYROCKETING POPULARITY combined with a lack of regulation has led to a landslide of misinformation and misunderstanding about the molecule. So let's set the record straight by dispelling some of the most common myths and replacing them with CBD facts.

MYTH #1:

CBD Is Not "Psychoactive"

Let's get this one straight right away. No, CBD will not get you high, so you won't end up giggly with a case of the munchies. You won't feel "zoned out" or "stoned." You won't get intoxicated or experience any of the mind-altering effects that you can get from smoking or ingesting sufficient amounts of CBD's sibling molecule in the cannabis plant, THC.

This, however, does not mean that CBD is not psychoactive. It most definitely is. CBD can have moderating effects on anxiety, depression, pain, appetite, and other brain activity, which by definition makes it psychoactive. That may sound like splitting hairs, but it's important to recognize that CBD is most definitely acting on your brain chemistry. When a clinically depressed patient takes a low dose of a CBD-rich sublingual spray or tincture and has a great day for the first time in a long time, it's apparent that CBD is a powerful mood-altering compound. Recognizing that CBD is indeed psychoactive is important for recognizing how the supplement is affecting you.

MYTH #2:

CBD Is Medicinal; THC Is Recreational

Because THC is "the high causer," people often dismiss it as "recreational," something to do at parties or a fun way to pass the time. But it's a lot more than that.

The FDA acknowledges that THC has clear medicinal benefits (which is why it is federally legal for doctors to prescribe it in its pure form as dronabinol (brand name Marinol), an antinausea compound and appetite booster. This synthetic form of THC is classified as a Schedule III pharmaceutical, a category reserved for drugs with little abuse potential. Yet, the cannabis plant, which is the only natural source of THC, continues to be federally classified as a dangerous Schedule I drug with no medical value. As we embrace CBD, it's worthwhile considering the value of legalizing cannabis, not just THC or CBD, on the federal level.

Project CBD refers to THC and CBD as "the power couple of cannabis therapeutics." They work best together. CBD and THC interact synergistically to amplify each other's curative qualities. CBD enhances THC's painkilling and anticancer properties, while decreasing or muting the high. CBD can also mitigate the adverse effects caused by too much THC, such as anxiety and rapid heartbeat. CBD and THC both stimulate neurogenesis, the creation of new brain cells, which has an antidepressant effect.[53] All of those benefits extend far beyond recreational use.

MYTH #3:

"Pure" CBD Isolate Is the Most Potent Form of CBD

As a culture, we tend to focus on the power of "active ingredients." We take vitamin and mineral supplements that concentrate a single molecule into a powerful pill. But very often, those single molecules actually work a lot better when they're combined with the others that they're found with in nature. For instance, beta-carotene, the antioxidant pigment found in carrots and colorful vegetables, is protective against free-radical damage when taken along with the other carotenoids and vitamins naturally found in those foods. But when isolated and taken as a single supplement, studies showed it could actually do more harm than good.

That's not saying that isolated CBD is dangerous or harmful, but it's a reminder that commercial supplement manufacturers don't generally know more than Mother Nature. Though our pharmaceutical-drug-oriented minds might automatically assume that isolated CBD is the most potent form you can find, the molecule (as mentioned previously) works best in synergy with other cannabis compounds.

Scientific studies have established that CBD and THC enhance each other's therapeutic effects. For example, British researchers conducting animal studies have reported that CBD increases the power of THC's anti-inflammatory properties in treating colitis.[54] Scientists at the California Pacific Medical Center in San Francisco determined that a combination of CBD and THC has a more potent antitumoral effect than either compound alone when tested on brain cancer and breast cancer cells in the lab.[55] Extensive clinical research has demonstrated that CBD combined with THC is more beneficial for neuropathic pain (pain caused by a malfunctioning nervous system) than either compound as a single molecule.

Plus, remember that cannabis contains several hundred compounds, including various flavonoids, aromatic terpenes, and many minor cannabinoids, in addition to THC and CBD. Each of these compounds has specific healing attributes, but when combined, they create what scientists refer to as the holistic entourage effect or ensemble effect, so that the therapeutic impact of the whole plant is greater than the sum of its single-molecule parts.

MYTH #4:

CBD Converts to THC in Your Stomach

It does not. But misleading headlines surrounding research a few years back raised concerns about the possible harmful side effects of CBD converting to THC in your stomach—an obvious problem for those who are concerned about drug testing or who are particularly sensitive to THC.

In 2016, the journal *Cannabis and Cannabinoid Research* published a paper suggesting that CBD converts to THC in the stomach. In the study, which was conducted in a laboratory setting (not on people), the researchers mixed CBD with acid designed to simulate the gastric fluid in your stomach. They found that a tiny amount of CBD degrades to psychotropic cannabinoids delta-8-THC and delta-9-THC. The researchers concluded, "The acidic environment during normal gastrointestinal transit can expose orally CBD-treated patients to levels of THC and other psychoactive cannabinoids that may exceed the threshold for a positive physiological response."[56] The researchers cautioned health-care providers against the oral use of CBD and recommended other delivery methods. In this case, unacknowledged commercial interests appeared to undermine scientific integrity, as the researchers were invloved with a business that sought to develop a transdermal delivery system for CBD.

Follow-up studies negated concerns about CBD turning into THC in the stomach. In a letter to the same journal in 2017, a different group of scientists asserted that "clinical data do not support this conclusion and recommendation, since even high doses of oral CBD do not cause psychological, psychomotor, cognitive, or physical effects that are characteristic for THC or cannabis rich in THC. . . . In addition, administration of CBD did not result in detectable THC blood concentrations. Thus, there is no reason to avoid oral use of CBD, which has been demonstrated to be a safe means of administration of CBD, even at very high doses."[57]

There have been extensive clinical trials demonstrating that ingested CBD—even doses above 600 mg—does not cause THC-like psychoactive effects (get you high). On the contrary, CBD in sufficient amounts can lessen or neutralize the THC high. In 2017, the World Health Organization issued a report that definitively asserted: "Simulated gastric fluid does not exactly replicate physiological conditions in the stomach [and] spontaneous conversion of CBD to delta-9-THC has not been demonstrated in humans undergoing CBD treatment."[58]

> Ingested CBD—even doses above 600 mg does not cause THC-like psychoactive effects.

MYTH #5:

CBD Is Fully Legal in the United States

Not quite, but the laws are evolving, and few people are being arrested for using CBD. The current legal quagmire is a result of our convoluted federal and state cannabis laws.

The 2018 Farm Bill legalized the cultivation of industrial hemp (defined as cannabis with no more that 0.3 percent THC) in the United States and removed derivatives of hemp, including CBD, from the purview of the Drug Enforcement Administration (DEA) and the Controlled Substances Act. But the federal Food and Drug Administration (FDA) has persisted in viewing CBD strictly as a pharmaceutical drug (Epidiolex) and maintains that it is illegal to sell hemp-derived CBD products as a dietary supplement. The DEA, meanwhile, retains jurisdiction over CBD derived from marijuana (cannabis with more than 0.3 percent THC), which is still prohibited under federal law.

Some states still restrict CBD purchase and possession to only those with a prescription. As of mid-2020, in some states like Idaho and South Dakota, CBD products were still considered illegal.[59] (See page 16 for more information on the legalities of CBD.)

You should also be cautious about flying with CBD. Though the TSA allows FDA-approved marijuana-based drugs and CBD produced from hemp with no more than 0.3 percent THC, if you're traveling in a state where trace amounts of THC are illegal and you have a full-spectrum product, TSA has the authority to contact local law enforcement officers.[60]

MYTH #6:

You Can't Fail a Drug Test on CBD

If you are taking a CBD isolate or broad-spectrum CBD product, which has all the THC removed in processing, you should not fail a standard workplace drug test, which looks for THC. (That's assuming that the CBD product is accurately labeled, which is often not the case.) But if you are taking full-spectrum CBD products, which may have up to 0.3 percent THC in them, beware. Though that is a miniscule amount, THC may accumulate in fat tissue with regular use, and it remains detectable in urine for days (or even weeks) after use.

If your job requires you to pass drug tests, it's very important to purchase your CBD products from a reputable supplier that guarantees it contains no THC. Remember, CBD products are unregulated and often mislabeled, so they may contain less CBD and more THC than claimed. Look for products from a company that can provide an independent third-party Certificate of Analysis that certifies their product was tested and contains the amount of CBD and THC listed on the label.

MYTH #7:

CBD Makes You Sleepy

Many people take CBD to help them sleep better, but it doesn't always make you sleepy, which is a good thing if you want to use it during times that you want to be fully awake. Actually, a small dose of CBD can make you feel more alert.

CBD produces what is called a *biphasic effect*, which means that low and high doses can produce opposite effects. So while moderate doses of CBD can be mildly energizing, higher doses of CBD can be sleep-promoting. For people with anxiety, CBD may help restore healthy sleep patterns by reducing their anxiety, so they don't toss and turn with worrying thoughts.

THC can also promote a good night's sleep perhaps even more effectively than CBD. That's also the case for myrcene, a terpene present in many cannabis varietals, which is known to have sedative and pain-killing properties. If you are using a full-spectrum CBD product, you may also be consuming small amounts of THC and myrcene, which can contribute to restful and rejuvenating sleep.

Some cannabis clinicians recommend that people start using CBD at home a few hours before bedtime. That way you can safely evaluate any side effects, and if it does make you feel drowsy, it won't interfere with your productivity (or safety if you're driving) during the day.

MYTH #8:

You'll Feel the Effects of CBD Right Away

Again, it depends. Some people feel the relaxing effects of a CBD-rich tincture under their tongue fairly quickly. Others may experience a more subtle effect that takes longer to materialize.

Depending on what you're taking CBD for, you may also need a higher or lower dose or a different form of the supplement to maxi-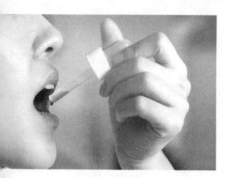mize the effect. There is no one-size-fits-all approach to CBD, so it may take some trial and error to see what works for you.

Generally speaking, if you try CBD and you feel absolutely nothing, don't just throw in the towel and assume it doesn't work. Instead, gradually increase your dosage and see if you notice a difference. Be patient and give it a few weeks. If you're getting blood tests under a doctor's supervision, compare the results before and after you start taking CBD. Check to see if your CBD regimen has improved your blood sugar levels and other indicators.

In the case of topical CBD, such as lotions used for muscle and joint pain and inflammation, the beneficial effects may appear more quickly. Some people report nearly instant relief. Others report that it just doesn't work for them. Again, you may need to experiment with products and dosages to get the desired effect.

MYTH #9:

You Need Clinically Proven Doses to Get Benefits

There is no one recommended dosage of CBD. When used as a prescription pharmaceutical, the dosage tends to be very high—ranging from 5 mg/kg per day to up to 20 mg/kg per day. That's the typical dosage range of Epidiolex for children with epilepsy, which translates to 340 to 1,360 mg per day for a 150-pound person. That's a huge dose, much more than most people would ever take using an unlicensed, hemp-derived CBD product (especially considering that CBD is not inexpensive). For serious diseases like Parkinson's, ALS, and chronic, debilitating pain, something approaching clinical doses of a CBD isolate might be in order. But when combined with THC or other cannabis components, the amount of CBD necessary for a therapeutic effect may be significantly less than the dosage recommended for Epidiolex.

> CBD isolates require higher doses to be effective than whole-plant CBD-rich oil extracts.

To assuage everyday aches and pains, take the edge off anxiety, or get a better night's rest, you can likely benefit from considerably lower doses. Manufacturers generally recommend between 10 and 50 mg of CBD per day depending on your body weight and severity of symptoms.

It's important to keep in mind that CBD isolates require higher doses to be effective than whole-plant CBD-rich oil extracts. Reports from medical cannabis clinicians and patients suggest that a synergistic combination of CBD, THC, and other cannabis components can be effective at low doses—sometimes as little as 2.5 mg CBD combined with a similar amount of THC.

But many people need a stronger dose to notice a difference in their health. Remember that low and high doses can produce opposite effects. So an excessive amount of CBD could actually be less effective therapeutically in some cases than a moderate dose. Chapter 9 can help you figure out what dose to start with.

MYTH #10:

All Types of CBD Products Work the Same Way

Far from it. Placing a few drops of a tincture under your tongue (taking CBD sublingually) will work faster—and require smaller doses to be effective—than taking CBD in a gummy or soft gel capsule. When you consume CBD in food, drink, or pill form, you need to wait for the digestive process to work, and you lose some active ingredients along the way. Vaping has also been a popular way to use CBD, because inhalation works nearly instantly and discretely. But vaping poor-quality, unlicensed, illicit CBD oil may lead to serious illness if it contains toxic fillers, so it's very important to make informed decisions about what to consume. See Chapter 7 for more information on different delivery methods.

MYTH #11:

CBD Has No Side Effects

As we'll discuss on page 182, the World Health Organization issued a statement that "there is no evidence of health-related problems associated with the use of pure CBD." That means they generally consider it safe. But that does not mean there are no side effects. It's important to remember that any substance that has the power to fix health problems may also have the power to cause side effects.

In the case of CBD, those unwanted side effects are generally pretty minimal: The most commonly reported ones are dry mouth and fatigue—and much depends on the quality of the CBD product one is consuming. More serious concerns arise if you're taking CBD in conjunction with other medications, especially if they're also metabolized by the same liver enzymes (as many are).

CBD can increase the levels of other medications, like blood thinners, in your blood, which can be dangerous. If you're taking other medications, you should check with your doctor before adding CBD to the mix. See Chapter 10 for more information.

MYTH #12:

All CBD Products Are Safe and Effective

Not even close. We'll take a deeper dive later in the book, but when buying CBD, it's important to know what to look for in terms of quality control. Hemp is a *bioaccumulator* that draws toxins from the soil, so products should be tested for safety and purity.

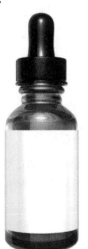

Currently, the FDA does not closely regulate the purity and/or safety of dietary supplements, so you cannot know for sure that the product you buy has active ingredients at the dose listed on the label. And there are quite a few questionable products on the market. In a recent study published in *the Journal of the American Medical Association,* researchers found that of 84 CBD products from 31 companies bought online, 26 percent of them contained less CBD than listed on the label. Only 30 percent of the products were accurately labeled. THC was found in 18 of the 84 products, despite not appearing on the label.[61]

It's important to find third-party-tested products from labs that are licensed and reputable. (See Chapter 8 for more information.)

2

CBD
for Health

I F YOU HAVE this book in your hands, chances are you are seeking relief from something (or more than one something) and have heard that CBD may help.

You are not alone. A 2019 *Consumer Reports* survey of more than 4,000 people found that 26 percent of Americans have tried CBD at least once in the past two years. Seven percent say they use it every day. The majority of responders said it helps with anxiety, joint pain, sleep, and a host of other issues.[1] There are many anecdotal accounts (a few of which you'll see throughout this book) of people having sometimes remarkable success treating diseases of all kinds with even small amounts of CBD.

It's possible, if not likely, that some of these people are experiencing a placebo effect. Usually used in scientific studies, a placebo is a fake treatment, like a sugar pill containing no medicine. Often, people given a placebo still feel better (even when they know it's not the real medicine) because the ritual of taking a pill triggers a healing response in the brain. But studies on animals and on human cells in the lab (which don't get the placebo effect) indicate that there's more than the placebo effect at work.[2,3]

Presently, there are only three conditions for which the FDA has approved CBD as a treatment. In June 2018, the FDA approved a CBD isolate drug called Epidiolex, which can reduce severe, largely untreatable seizures in children with two kinds of epilepsy (Dravet's syndrome and Lennox-Gastaut syndrome).[4] In August 2020, the FDA approved the use of Epidiolex to also treat seizures in patients with tuberous sclerosis complex, a genetic disorder characterized by benign tumors in the brain, kidneys, and other organs.[5] Another cannabinoid-based drug called Sativex, consisting of a mixture of CBD and THC, has been approved to treat pain and spasticity in multiple sclerosis patients in more than two dozen countries but not in the United States.

Unfortunately, clinical research still lags behind the public's appetite for CBD knowledge. As mentioned previously, because CBD is derived from hemp—a type of cannabis that is a botanical cousin to marijuana—it's been difficult, and often illegal, to conduct clinical research. So gold-standard, double-blind, randomized clinical trials on real people are still few and far between. The vast majority of current CBD research consists mainly of preclinical studies (petri dish and animal research that takes place before human studies can be done) that focus on single-molecule cannabinoids. Though it's all worth noting and often promising, preclinical studies are not necessarily applicable to human experience. Medical knowledge is limited by those constraints.

But that doesn't mean we don't have a growing (and convincing) body of research on CBD. As we described earlier, CBD can help us rebalance our innate endocannabinoid system, taming the chronic stress and systemic inflammation that underlie a wide range of diseases and disorders. As scientists learn more about this critical system and how cannabinoids like CBD interact with it, they are developing a clearer picture of how CBD can help us. So while it's always wise to maintain healthy skepticism when something is touted as a "cure-all," there are reasons to be optimistic about the future of CBD for health and wellness.

We've compiled an A–Z list of some of the diseases and health disorders that CBD may benefit as a preventive measure and/or as a treatment. In this section, you'll get a snapshot of the current science for each. This is by no means a comprehensive list. As research continues apace on CBD's effects on the human body, other conditions may be added. Refer to ProjectCBD.org for updates. The pages that follow focus on some of the most common health issues for which people are turning to CBD.

Acne and Skin Conditions

YOUR SKIN IS a complex, multifunctional, protective barrier for your body. It's also the largest and heaviest organ we carry around—about one-seventh of our total body's weight, or 8 to 22 pounds on average—with a surface area of about 2 square yards.

Though we think of it as a single fleshy wrap around our body, our skin is actually comprised of three layers. The outermost, called the *epidermis*, is like a fortress wall, a strong yet flexible barrier made up of constantly renewing skin cells. Below the *epidermis* is the *dermis*, which houses a complex collection of nerves and capillaries. And then there's the deepest layer, known as the hypodermis, which attaches the skin to the rest of the body. Vitamin D and other essential hormones are synthesized in the hypodermis.[6]

Your skin cells also house CB_1 and CB_2 cannabinoid receptors, which, when signaling, can help promote healthy skin renewal and barrier function, according to a 2019 study conducted by a team of Hungarian researchers from the University of Debrecen.[7]

A recent report by German scientists in *Experimental Dermatology* concluded that if the skin's endocannabinoid signaling is thrown out of balance, it may pave the way for various skin diseases and conditions, including:

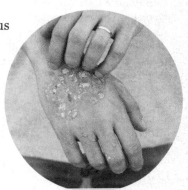

- atopic dermatitis
- allergic contact dermatitis
- acne
- seborrhea
- psoriasis
- itching
- pain
- hair growth disorders
- systemic sclerosis

It may also delay wound healing.[8]

Based on these findings, it's reasonable to speculate that a topically applied CBD-infused cream or salve may prevent and treat a variety of skin conditions. Specific studies on acne and psoriasis have shown some promise.

In a 2014 study, Hungarian scientists described CBD as a potent "universal" anti-acne agent after they showed that the cannabinoid prevents skin cells from producing too much sebum, the oil that protects our skin. Sebum can trigger acne when it's trapped with dirt inside our pores. CBD also set off an anti-inflammatory reaction in the cells and prevented them from activating proteins that may cause acne.[9]

Another study on skin samples in the lab found that cannabinoid receptors in the skin have the ability to reduce excess skin growth. In theory, an effective remedy for excess skin cell production could help with dermatitis and psoriasis, two common inflammatory conditions that speed up the life cycle of skin cells and cause a buildup of cells on the surface of the skin, creating red, itchy, sometimes painful patches. A small 2019 study published in *Clinical Therapeutics* reported that CBD ointment used for three months significantly improved symptoms of psoriasis and atopic dermatitis.[10]

It may even be useful against serious antibiotic-resistant infections like methicillin-resistant *Staphylococcus aureus*, or MRSA, a highly contagious, potentially fatal bacterial skin infection commonly associated with hospitalized people with compromised immune systems.[11] MRSA has also cropped up in locker rooms, gyms, daycare facilities, and other places people congregate.

A 2008 study published by the American Chemical Society in the *Journal of Natural Products* reported that CBD and another cannabis compound called *cannabigerol* (CBG) "showed potent activity against a variety of MRSA strains."[12] Three other plant cannabinoids—THC, cannabinol (CBN), and cannabichromene (CBC)—also showed encouraging results in preclinical research.

The American Chemical Society journal concluded: "Given the availability of C. *sativa* strains producing high concentrations of nonpsychotropic cannabinoids, [the cannabis] plant represents an interesting source of antibacterial agents to address the problem of multidrug resistance in MRSA and other pathogenic bacteria. This issue has enormous clinical implications, since MRSA is spreading throughout the world and, in the United States, currently accounts for more deaths each year than AIDS. Although the use of cannabinoids as systemic antibacterial agents awaits rigorous clinical trials...their topical application to reduce skin colonization by MRSA seems promising."[13]

Addictions and Alcoholism

A S AN ANTI-INFLAMMATORY that helps quell anxiety and boosts the release of your body's natural pain blockers, CBD can go a long way in making you feel good. It's also nonaddictive and does not cause withdrawal symptoms if or when you stop using it.[14] This means that for some people, the molecule could be a pain-relieving alternative to habit-forming opioid drugs.

CBD may also help people overcome their current addictions due to its toning effects on the endocannabinoid system, which in turn impacts memory, or more specifically our ability to forget.[15,16] Many of our cravings are grounded in how our brain remembers an experience (after all, you wouldn't crave a drink if you've never had one). As anyone who has ever tried to cut back or quit an addictive substance like nicotine or alcohol knows, it's exponentially harder to avoid relapsing when exposed to familiar environmental cues associated with past addictive behavior, whether at home or work settings or, for example, when bombarded by a steady stream of beer commercials during a football game.

When someone who has taken drugs or alcohol is exposed to a drug- or alcohol-related environmental cue, it can trigger a yearning for that experience. CBD may step in and interfere with cue-induced memories to reduce future cravings. It's been successful in animal studies, as reported in the *Journal of Addiction Biology* in 2017.[17] Rats addicted to heroin lost their attraction to it after being treated with CBD.[18]

Similarly, a 2009 paper demonstrated that CBD suppresses the cues or triggers associated with heroin.[19] By interacting with memory systems in the brain, CBD helps to ease compulsions to use opioids. Researchers led by Yasmin Hurd, PhD, at Mount Sinai in New York have published several papers on these topics, the most recent being a clinical trial of CBD for reducing relapse to heroin. Taking high doses of a pure CBD isolate (400 mg–800 mg) dramatically reduced the likelihood that participants would take heroin when triggered by the things they associated with it. Simultaneously, it ameliorated the extreme anxiety and discomfort that typically occur during withdrawal. And the positive effects lingered. After dosing CBD for three days, the participants experienced relief for up to a week, similar to what has been seen in laboratory and animal studies.

This research suggests that CBD may aid in unlearning the habits surrounding addiction that can lead to cravings and relapse well after withdrawal has subsided. CBD also may help restore healthy endocannabinoid system activity, which research shows is disrupted by substance abuse.

In a 2019 study, a team of Spanish researchers concluded: "Substance abuse causes a disruption in the synaptic plasticity of the brain circuits involved in addiction, with the alteration of normal endocannabinoid activity playing a prominent role. This facilitates abnormal changes in the brain and the development of the addictive behaviours that characterise substance use disorders."[20] In other words, substance abuse wreaks havoc on the endocannabinoid system, which can reinforce an addictive cycle.

Researchers at the University of Madrid showed that binge drinking in rats lowers endocannabinoid activity and reduces neurogenesis, the growth of new brain cells, in the hippocampus region of the brain.[21] Other studies show that stimulating hippocampal neurogenesis, which CBD is known to do, may help treat alcohol addiction and depression.[22, 23]

Project CBD's extensive 2019 survey, which included 3,506 people spanning the globe, representing 58 different countries, yielded hopeful results. The majority of those using CBD to tame their substance abuse issues reported being addicted to alcohol (68 percent), tobacco (38 percent), and/or opiates (36 percent). A smaller percent reported being addicted to benzodiazepines, amphetamines, cocaine, sleeping medications, ketamine, food, sugar, caffeine, and high-THC cannabis. Participants taking CBD for addiction were very likely to report that they were also taking CBD for mood issues (78 percent), pain (69 percent), sleep problems (58 percent), and/or PTSD (30 percent).

The survey also found that about 50 percent said they stopped using alcohol and 45 percent used less after using CBD. It was comparatively less helpful as a smoking cessation aid. Twenty-four percent of tobacco users experienced no change, and 4 percent reported using more tobacco after introducing CBD.[24]

Perhaps most exciting is the research showing that CBD and cannabis can be effective in breaking an addiction to opioids.[25] Observational studies (where researchers collect data based on what is seen and heard) have reported that many people voluntarily decrease the amount of opioids they are using—or go off opioids completely—when

> CBD may help treat alcohol addiction and depression.

they use them in conjunction with cannabis. And animal and laboratory studies suggest that cannabis and CBD may reduce the risk of relapse.[26]

For instance, a 2016 Israeli study of 176 opioid-using adults found that opioid use was reduced by 44 percent after they began smoking cannabis or eating cannabis-infused cookies.[27] Similarly, in a survey of more than 1,000 of his patients, Dr. Dustin Sulak, DO, the founder and director of Integr8 Health, a network of holistic health clinics specializing in cannabis therapeutics, found that many stopped using opioids completely after starting cannabis.[28] Of those patients, "73 percent stayed off opioids for over a year and an additional 39 percent had reduced their dose of opioids.... Forty-seven percent reported a reduction in pain greater than 40 percent—that's considered very effective in the medical literature. Eighty percent reported improved function; and 87 percent reported improvement in their quality of life," he says.

If you're dealing with chronic pain and/or are already taking pain medications like opioids for it, it may be worth talking with your doctor about combining CBD with other medications. CBD may help you manage your pain while

69

reducing your opioid dosage and minimizing withdrawal symptoms as you wean yourself away from those powerful prescription pharmaceuticals.

Anxiety

WHEN THE COVID-19 crisis began in March 2020, people started stockpiling essentials like cleaning products, toilet paper, and yes, CBD. An April 2020 Brightfield Group survey of consumers who have used CBD in the past 12 months found that nearly 50 percent had stocked up or planned to stock up on CBD products.[29, 30]

Why stockpile CBD? Because one of the most popular uses of the cannabinoid is to calm anxiety, and a global pandemic creates massive amounts of anxiety and exacerbates anxiety disorders, like obsessive-compulsive disorder (OCD), post-traumatic stress disorder (PTSD), phobias, and panic disorder. If you've ever suffered from anxiety, you know the symptoms all too well: Nervousness, tension, panic, a sense of doom, increased heart rate, sweating, and fatigue make it difficult to concentrate on anything else. Almost one in three adults in the United States experiences an anxiety disorder at some time in their lives.[31]

When you consider that one of your endocannabinoid system's primary responsibilities is to regulate fear and anxiety and to help us manage stress, it's no surprise that using CBD can help you manage stress-related conditions like anxiety. As explained in Chapter 2, CBD delays the "reuptake" and breakdown of the bliss molecule anandamide, so you have more of the mood-improving cannabinoid in your system. In addition, CBD directly activates a serotonin receptor known as 5-HTIA, which causes an antianxiety effect. It also makes it easier for GABA receptors to bind with your body's own GABA molecules, which amplifies their natural calming effect. Finally, animal studies suggest that CBD's brain-building benefits may also help protect against anxiety-related depression by boosting the growth of brain cells

"I Tried It"

Emily Wilson, 31,
Athens, Greece

EMILY WILSON, a 31-year-old British aid worker living in Greece, was working as an education coordinator at a refugee camp on the outskirts of Athens, where 2,800 displaced persons from countries like Syria, Afghanistan, Iraq, and Iran live side by side in converted shipping containers, many still suffering from severe trauma.

With limited resources, Emily was often left feeling stressed and frustrated by the limitations of the work she could do. After two years working at the refugee camp, her naturally buoyant and positive nature was no longer a protection against the physical and mental strain she endured on a daily basis.

Emily shared her experience with journalist Mary Biles, a Project CBD contributing writer. "I remember a few times," Emily recounted, "where I'd just be walking and I'd start to think about work and my chest would tighten and I'd have to start taking deep breaths because my chest was tightening so much and my eyes were watering like I was crying. But it was tears of frustration and tears of panic. This happened about once or twice a week for about three or four weeks until I realized there was something really wrong. It was so crippling that I didn't go to work because I couldn't get out of bed."

Emily started taking full-spectrum CBD oil, and after gradually building up the dose from one drop to three drops, three times a day, she started to feel her anxiety levels subside.

"I think the major benefit of it for me," says Emily, "was it prevented the anxiety from becoming all-encompassing. It didn't take away the problems, but meant that they were there, I acknowledged them, I knew that I had to work through them, but they weren't in my chest, they weren't in my throat, and weren't stopping me doing things. So there was a distance from them. I also felt a deep sense of calm and a deep sense of, OK, well, everything can be solved."[33]

in the hippocampus, the area of the brain that regulates emotion, motivation, learning, and memory.[32]

Research on the use of CBD for anxiety and panic disorders has been somewhat mixed but mostly promising. One 2015 analysis of 49 studies published in the journal *Neurotherapeutics* concluded that scientific evidence supports CBD as a viable treatment for a variety of anxiety disorders, including panic disorder, generalized anxiety disorder, obsessive-compulsive disorder, and social anxiety disorder.

CBD may not only calm anxiety, making you feel more relaxed, but also may change the way your brain responds to anxiety-producing stimuli.[34]

The overall body of research regarding CBD and general anxiety leans in a positive direction. The researchers involved in the 2015 *Neurotherapeutics* analysis reported that doses of CBD isolate in the range of 300 mg to 600 mg reduced experimentally induced anxiety.

In another study published in the *Journal of Psychopharmacology*, researchers gave a group of people with social anxiety disorder either 400 mg of CBD or a placebo capsule, then scanned their brain activity and asked them to rate their anxiety levels. At a later date, they had the volunteers return and repeat the test, this time switching who got the dummy pills and who got the CBD supplements. Compared to the times they were given placebos, the participants enjoyed significantly lower feelings of anxiety, and their brain scans showed altered activity in the limbic area, which is instrumental in regulating emotions and anxiety, after they took CBD.[35]

Brazilian scientists examined the effects of CBD on social anxiety disorder, a common anxiety condition that causes people to experience intense fear of being judged or rejected in social situations. Their findings were published in *Neuropsychopharmacology*. The researchers gave 24 adults with social anxiety disorder either 600 mg of CBD or a placebo capsule before having them perform a public speaking test (which is enough to give anyone anxiety). Those who got the CBD experienced significantly less anxiety, cognitive impairment, and negative feelings about themselves before performing the test than did those participants who had received a placebo pill. Remarkably, the CBD-taking public speakers' anxiety before the test was similar to a group of healthy adults who did not have social anxiety disorder. The volunteers who didn't get CBD, by contrast, experienced significantly higher levels of anxiety, cognitive impairment, and discomfort.[36]

Of course, you can be anxious and have episodes of anxiety without being diagnosed with an anxiety disorder. Plenty of people use CBD to alleviate low levels of everyday anxiety as well. Anecdotally, many people say they feel relief from their anxiety at far lower doses than those used in scientific studies.

Respondents to Project CBD's 2019 survey feel largely the same. Almost 90 percent of participants using CBD for a mood disorder reported that they had anxiety. CBD appeared to perform especially well at calming feelings of nervousness: 92 percent of participants experienced some relief from this symptom, and 68 percent reported that feelings

> Participants enjoyed significantly lower feelings of anxiety.

of nervousness were "much better" with CBD. CBD also performed well at relieving panic attacks, reducing mood swings, and quelling feelings of agitation, irritability, and sadness.

CBD was less effective at mitigating difficulties in concentrating, a lack of interest in activities, and anxiety-related digestive upset; almost a fifth of people reported no change in these symptoms. Three percent of people using CBD for a mood disorder reported that the ability to concentrate actually worsened with CBD. But more often than not, consumers indicate that CBD in moderate doses improves concentration.[37]

When it comes to taking CBD for anxiety and anxiety-related conditions, it's important to remember that CBD works on a bell-shaped curve, so while a moderate dose may ease anxiety, too-high doses may be less effective or make things worse.

Case in point, in a study published in the *Journal of Psychopharmacology*, London researchers tested CBD on 32 people who suffered from anxiety and paranoia.[38] The researchers immersed the participants in a virtual reality simulation of being on a London Underground train. The virtual trek made about 40 percent of participants feel paranoid and threatened. Then the researchers gave the group either 600 mg of CBD isolate or a dummy pill and sent them back into the simulation. The high doses of CBD were not helpful in this experiment. In fact, the people given CBD tended to be more anxious than their placebo-treated counterparts.

Another study published in the *Brazilian Journal of Psychiatry* found that CBD might lose its effect when the dose is too large, with 300 mg of pure CBD seeming to be a sweet spot for dosing for social anxiety.[39]

As of mid-2020, a number of clinical trials to study the effectiveness of CBD for anxiety were just getting started, including one study using 25 mg of full-spectrum CBD soft gel capsules over a period of 12 weeks; and a phase II clinical trial evaluating the efficacy of CBD for social anxiety, which will also measure changes in endocannabinoid levels.[40] And a Harvard Medical School research project will also compare whole-plant and single-extract CBD solutions for anxiety.

Harvard University scientist Staci Gruber, PhD, says preliminary data "suggests significant improvement following four weeks of treatment when compared to baseline.... Specifically, findings suggest that the use of a custom-formulated, whole plant-derived high CBD sublingual tincture results in less severe anxiety and fewer anxiety-related symptoms."[41]

Autism

THE NUMBER OF children diagnosed with autism spectrum disorders (ASD) worldwide has tripled in the past 30 years. Now there's undeniable evidence that endocannabinoid system dysregulation is involved and that some people with ASD have low endocannabinoid system tone.

In 2019, in a review paper titled "Endocannabinoid system involvement in autism spectrum disorder: An overview with potential therapeutic applications," researchers concluded: "Recent evidence highlights a strong involvement of the EC system in the

pathophysiology of some neuropsychiatric disorders and of ASD....
Additionally, evidence from the literature indicates that CBD may
alleviate many conditions co-occurring with ASD, such as seizures,
gastrointestinal problems, anxiety and depression,
attention deficit, and sleep problems."[42]

Parents seem to agree. In 2019, Israeli
researchers surveyed the parents of 53
children and young adults, ages 4 to 22,
who were receiving oral drops of CBD
oil for an average of 66 days.[43] Self-harm
and rage attacks improved in nearly 68
percent, hyperactivity improved in 68
percent, 71 percent slept better, and 47 percent had less anxiety. In some cases, symptoms
worsened: 24 percent seemed to become more anxious, for instance.
Otherwise, the outcomes were mostly positive, and the adverse side
effects, mostly changes in appetite and feeling sleepy, were mild.

Another study published in *Nature* in 2019 analyzed data from 188
children with ASD who were treated with medical cannabis—mostly
CBD-rich cannabis oil—between 2015 and 2017. After six months
of treatment, just under a third of participants reported significant
improvements and more than half reported moderate improvements,
according to quality of life questionnaires that measured mood and
the ability to function independently.[44]

Of course, more research is needed to provide more concrete recommendations, but in the meantime, it's worth a conversation with
a practitioner who is well-versed in CBD. In some cases, children can
have remarkable improvement with very small doses, says Bonni
Goldstein, MD, author of *Cannabis Is Medicine* and medical director
of Canna-Centers, a California-based medical practice devoted to
educating patients about the use of cannabis for serious and chronic
medical conditions.

"I had a patient, a little boy, come in with autism, and the parents were desperate. So they tried a little bit—and I mean a really little bit of CBD—before they came into my office, and they told me that after one week on that very low dose, the teacher had already noticed the child was doing better. The teacher did not know he was on CBD oil. But she made like a beeline for the mom one day at the end of school and said, 'Okay what's going on? What's different?' At that tiny dose, like about 4 or 5 milligrams, they were seeing this incredible benefit in this child."[45]

On the other side of the spectrum, she also sees patients who require much higher doses, and nobody can really say why, because CBD works on the cellular level and it's not easy to measure. "There's no way to tell by somebody's size or level of illness exactly what's going to fit them. You're not going to know until you try and see," Goldstein says.

Bone Health

CBD MADE BONE health headlines in 2015, when a team of Israeli researchers reported in the *Journal of Bone and Mineral Research* that the cannabinoid significantly helped heal bone fractures.

The study, conducted on rats with fractured femurs, found that CBD "markedly enhanced the healing process" after just eight weeks. CBD not only spurs the process of new bone-cell formation, but also makes the bones stronger during healing. In the experiment, the bones of rats treated with CBD were 35 to 50 percent stronger than those not treated with CBD during the healing period—decreasing the risk of refracturing the bone.[46]

In earlier research, the same team had discovered that cannabinoid receptors within our bodies stimulate bone formation and inhibit bone loss, which means they have the potential to combat bone-related diseases, such as osteoporosis, in which the density of the bone is reduced, making it fragile and easier to break.

When the endocannabinoid system becomes dysregulated, you can end up with more osteoblasts (the cells that break down bone) than osteoclasts (the cells that build it back up). Cannabinoids facilitate the process of bone metabolism—the cycle in which old bone material is replaced by new, which is crucial to maintaining strong, healthy bones over time.

CBD has also been shown to block an enzyme that destroys bone-building compounds in the body, reducing the risk of age-related bone diseases like osteoporosis and osteoarthritis. In both of those diseases, the body is no longer creating sufficient amounts of new bone and cartilage cells.

Cancer

W E TEND TO think of cancer as a single disease, but it's actually the name given to a collection of related diseases. In all types of cancer, some of your body's cells begin to divide without stopping and spread into surrounding tissues. Symptoms vary widely based on the type of cancer but frequently include pain, fatigue, nausea, and unexplained weight loss. Almost 40 percent of people will get a cancer diagnosis in their life.[47]

There is a growing body of evidence that shows cannabinoids can slow cancer growth, inhibit the formation of new blood cells that feed a tumor, and help manage pain, fatigue, nausea, and other side effects associated with this dreadful disease. A 2005 report published in *Mini-Reviews in Medicinal Chemistry* went so far as to state that cannabinoids "represent a new class of anticancer drugs."[48]

In some cases, CBD may be able to fight cancer by switching off key genes that contribute to the disease. In a study published in 2011 in the journal *Breast Cancer Research and Treatment*, CBD researcher Sean McAllister, PhD, and his coworkers at the California Pacific

Medical Center in San Francisco published a detailed account of how cannabidiol kills breast cancer cells and destroys malignant tumors by switching off expression of the ID-1 gene, a protein that appears to play a role as a cancer cell conductor.[49]

The ID-1 gene is active while cells are developing in the womb, but after we're born, it turns off and is supposed to stay off. But in certain breast cancers and several other types of metastatic cancer, the ID-1 gene becomes active again, paving the way for malignant cells to invade and metastasize, or spread. "Dozens of aggressive cancers express this gene," McAllister explained. Though the ID-1 gene is not the sole "cause" of these cancers and is not a factor in the majority of cancers, silencing it may offer one avenue of treatment for those cancers that are related to the ID-1 gene.

CBD appears to be beneficial in the fight against glioblastoma multiforme (a particularly aggressive form of brain cancer). A 2018 medical case report by Dra. Paula Dall'Stella, a neuro-oncologist with Sirio Libanes Hospital in São Paulo, Brazil, documented the antitumoral effects of CBD in two patients with glioblastoma multiforme that was resistant to other therapies. Before and after MRI scans showed "a marked remission...not commonly observed in patients only treated with conventional modalities...that could impact survival."[50]

A 2019 literature review of brain cancer case studies published in *Anticancer Research* reported that CBD did indeed positively impact survival among people diagnosed with these malignant brain tumors, which have a median survival rate of about 14 to 16 months. The study included case studies of a total of nine people with brain tumors who were given a daily dose of 400 mg of CBD along with their usual treatments. At the time of the study publication, all but one were still alive with an average survival time of 22.3 months, which is longer than typically expected.[51]

In April 2020, Colorado State University researchers studying human and canine brain cancer cells found that CBD isolate worked by slowing cancer cell growth and had toxic effects on glioblastoma cells.

"Further research and treatment options are urgently needed for patients afflicted by brain cancer," said Chase Gross, a student in the DVM/MS program at Colorado State University. "Our work shows that CBD has the potential to provide an effective, synergistic glioblastoma therapy option and that it should continue to be vigorously studied."[52]

The antitumor benefits extend to myriad types of cancer beyond the brain. A 2020 paper published by a team of scientists from the University of Porto, Portugal, concluded that "the anti-cancer properties of CBD have also been demonstrated by several pre-clinical studies in different types of tumour cells."[53]

> CBD appears to be beneficial in the fight against glioblastoma multiforme.

As mentioned in Chapter 3, one way CBD can help fight cancer is by deactivating the orphan receptor GPR55. A 2010 study by researchers at the Chinese Academy of Scientists reported that GPR55 activation promotes the proliferation of cancer cells.[54] By blocking the GPR55 receptor, CBD keeps it from signaling, which may help prevent cancer cells from multiplying.

Laboratory research also shows that CBD can make tumors shrink by activating a nuclear receptor known as PPAR-gamma, which can keep cancer cells from reproducing so quickly.[55] And a 2014 study published in *Phytomedicine* showed that a CBD-rich cannabis extract stopped the spread of colorectal cancer cells in mice.[56]

McAllister's lab also analyzed how CBD works in combination with first-line chemotherapy agents. His animal research found that CBD acts synergistically with some anticancer pharmaceuticals like Taxotere and bicalutamide, enhancing their impact.[57] Unlike FDA-approved chemotherapy agents, CBD doesn't harm healthy cells near the tumor.[58, 59]

An Interview with a Medical Cannabis Specialist

Bonni Goldstein, MD

Though mainstream medical science has been lagging behind in terms of cannabinoids and cancer, frontline doctors have been seeing remarkable results for some time. Martin A. Lee of Project CBD interviewed Bonni Goldstein, MD, medical director of Canna-Centers, a California-based medical practice devoted to educating patients about the use of cannabis for serious and chronic medical conditions and author of *Cannabis Is Medicine*. This edited conversation shows how CBD is helping cancer patients—sometimes with remarkable positive results—in the real world.[60]

Project CBD: *Can you share an inspiring story of a case that you've been involved with recently?*

Goldstein: I recently had a young woman come to me, a teenager, who had very advanced bone cancer called osteosarcoma. Her cancer was so advanced that it was actually kind of popping out of the bones through the skin in her legs. She also had a very large metastatic tumor in her lungs that was requiring her to be on oxygen. She was on pain pills. She came to my office in a wheelchair.

In the literature, there's an article on mice that shows that a combination of cannabis plus a particular chemotherapy drug is pretty good at cancer killing, when separately you may not get there. So, we put her on pretty high doses of a combination of CBG (cannabigerol), THC, and CBD. In just six months' time, her PET scan is not showing any cancer lighting up. The pulmonary tumor, which started off at around 12 centimeters, has shrunk by about 85 percent. She's out of the wheelchair. She's off oxygen. She's off pain medicine. She was able to go back to school in September. And she even made a trip to Colorado to go visit some family and friends. It's been really an amazing journey.

Project CBD: *You speak of using both conventional chemotherapy and cannabis oil together. Can you expound upon that a little bit?*

Goldstein: We don't have the ability to do clinical trials. So, until we know better, what I say, especially with pediatric cancers, you're going to throw everything you can. There are a handful of studies that look at cannabis plus some of the chemotherapeutic agents in terms of either cancer killing or in terms of cannabis mitigating some of the side effects of these very toxic medications. And so, when a patient comes in who's on some traditional chemotherapy, I always make sure I do a review of the science and the literature to make sure that we know we're not negating them. There's research now that's coming out of a pharmaceutical company in Great Britain for a very dangerous and deadly cancer of the brain called glioblastoma multiforme. Most people may know that as the tumor that Senator John McCain had.

Project CBD: *It's pretty much always fatal.*

Goldstein: Yes, after five years maybe 15 percent of people, if that, are alive. There's some evidence that these cancers are very sensitive to cannabinoids. One report shows that at the end of one year that 83 percent of patients who got the combination of CBD, THC, and chemo were still alive. Whereas the patients that got chemo alone, 53 percent were alive. Again, it's a small group, I think 20 patients. But there's certainly something there that is statistically significant. Not to mention that those patients taking THC and CBD seem to have a decent quality of life. It's not like we're adding on more toxic chemicals.

I had a parent that came in who said, "My doctor told me I should not give cannabis, specifically CBD, to my son with leukemia because they don't know long-term what it will do to his brain." Well, I know what chemotherapy does to children. About 60 to 70 percent of children who survive pediatric cancer have significant medical conditions that they have to deal with the rest of their lives. I've had patients who survive cancer and then only continue with cannabis, they are taken off chemo, they live a great quality of life. It's amazing.

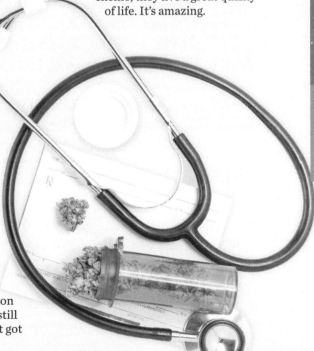

CBD may also help alleviate the symptoms of cancer and the miserable side effects of cancer treatment like chemotherapy. In Project CBD's 2019 survey, among people taking CBD for cancer, CBD was most helpful with ameliorating nausea and vomiting. Many participants also found it helpful for appetite, neuropathy (numbness or tingling), and weakness.

Cannabinoids like CBD may also provide another, nonaddictive, avenue for pain management in people with cancer.[61] Canada approved Sativex (an oromucosal spray that contains nearly equal parts THC and CBD) for the treatment of intractable cancer pain in 2007, and two dozen other countries have since authorized the use of Sativex for treating neuropathic pain and spasticity. [62]

Overall, CBD may be an important ally in the fight against cancer, helping to prevent and treat the disease, alleviate cancer symptoms, and/or lessen the severity of cancer treatment side effects like nausea.[63, 64] Research finds that CBD along with THC can make chemotherapy more effective, thereby reducing the amount of chemo necessary. Keep in mind that cannabinoids can inhibit enzymes like CYP2D6 and CYP3A4, which are responsible for metabolizing chemotherapy drugs.[65] By inhibiting those enzymes, it's possible to end up with more chemotherapy drugs in your system than the intended dose. That's why it's important that you work with your doctor if you want to use CBD-rich cannabis oil while undergoing chemo for cancer.

Chronic Pain

PAIN IS PHYSICAL suffering or discomfort typically caused by inflammatory conditions like arthritis, diseases like cancer, or an injury. When your pain lasts more than 12 weeks, it's considered chronic. But as anyone with chronic pain knows, it can persist for several months or even years. Twenty percent of the world's population suffers from chronic pain. About 60 percent of people suffering from chronic pain are women. Opioids are the most common treatment for chronic pain, even though substantial research shows that they are not effective.[66]

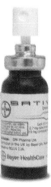

The endocannabinoid system regulates how we process pain and regulates pain signaling in the central nervous system. It's of little surprise then that cannabis has a long history as a pain reliever with doctors using it on their patients dating back to 2,700 BC in China.[67] In modern times, a 1999 Institutes of Medicine report concluded that "cannabinoids likely have a natural role in pain modulation." In 2005, Sativex (an oromucosal spray that contains equal parts THC and CBD) was approved in Canada for the treatment of neuropathic pain (shooting or burning pain caused by nerve damage or disease) associated with multiple sclerosis; later, it was approved to treat intractable cancer pain.[68]

Two dozen other countries subsequently approved Sativex as a treatment for chronic pain and spasticity. In 2018, researchers confirmed that the CBD/THC sublingual spray not only eased

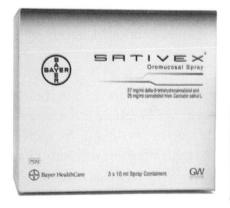

Sativex

"I Tried It"

Laurie Maxson, 65,
Colorado Springs,
Colorado

ABOUT FOUR years ago, Laurie Maxson, then 61, began to find it challenging to complete even the simplest tasks in the morning. "I started experiencing a lot of pain in my hands and feet and difficulty moving my fingers," says the retired school administrator from Colorado Springs, Colorado. "It was hard throughout the day but worst when I first woke up. I couldn't even grip a toothbrush."

Maxson scheduled an appointment with her doctor, who performed a physical exam and a series of blood tests. Soon, she had a diagnosis. "My numbers indicated that I had a moderate to severe case of rheumatoid arthritis," she says.

An autoimmune disorder, rheumatoid arthritis causes painful inflammation of the lining of the joints. It can often take sufferers multiple tries to find the right treatment. Maxson started a series of different medications but couldn't tolerate the side effects, which included extreme fatigue, nausea, and itching. She finally found relief with monthly infusions of a biologic

pain in people with multiple sclerosis, but also improved their pain sensitivity to cold temperatures.[69]

As with most conditions (and the success of pharmaceuticals like Sativex shows), CBD works best in concert with THC (and the rest of the cannabis entourage) for chronic pain relief. Dosage is key. In rare cases, THC-heavy cannabis can actually worsen pain, while a moderate dose of balanced cannabis, with a 1:1 ratio of CBD to THC, decreases pain.

To date, there have been no clinical trials on the efficacy of CBD alone for pain, though that is set to change. In 2020, Canadian researchers were readying to launch a pilot study to investigate the effectiveness of CBD oil on post-operative pain following knee replacement surgery.[71] Though the United States has been slow to recognize CBD-based medicine in the treatment of pain (Sativex is still not approved for use in the United States), pain is one of the areas of cannabinoid research sponsored by the National Institutes medication that blocks inflammation-causing substances.

Then she decided to set her sights higher. "I was good," she says. "But I wanted to be even better. And I wanted to be participating myself in my own health." She changed her diet, cutting way back on sugar, eating more plant-based foods and less red meat, and choosing organic fruits and vegetables at the market. And, scouring websites and blogs where people shared their experiences living with arthritis, Maxson began reading accounts of people who had been helped by CBD.

After careful research, Maxon decided to try a CBD tincture from hemp plants grown locally, which had been certified by a third-party lab to be free of heavy metals, pesticides, residual solvents, and microbes. Today, after several months of taking CBD daily, Maxson says, "I just feel like everything is working a little bit better and a little bit quicker. It's like oiling up a machine." Though she's had to give up the intense circuit-training workouts she once followed, she's back to exercising again, taking mat Pilates classes several times a week and walking regularly. "I realize that I have a chronic disease that affects my autoimmune system," Maxson says, "and I'm trying to do everything I can to live the best life I can. CBD is a piece of that."[70]

of Health, which has dedicated a modest three million dollars for cannabinoid pain studies.

CBD may help ease flare-ups and break the cycle of chronic pain in a few ways. For one, the cannabinoid boosts anxiety-calming serotonin (5HT1A) receptor activity, which may reduce pain signals. It also increases levels of anandamide, the "runner's high" cannabinoid, which binds to your CB1 receptors and blocks pain signaling and the emotional processing of those pain signals; this may reduce the amount of discomfort a person experiences.[72]

Board-certified neurologist Ethan Russo, MD, director of CReDO Science, has also theorized that common types of pain, such as migraine, fibromyalgia, and certain types of nerve pain, are the result of endocannabinoid deficiency, so logically improving endocannabinoid tone could reduce pain in those conditions.[73]

CBD is also a known anti-inflammatory, which makes it particularly useful for pain related to inflammatory conditions like arthritis.

A 2017 animal study published in the journal *Pain* concluded that CBD could decrease joint inflammation and protect the nerves from inflammatory damage. In this way, CBD can help prevent osteoarthritis pain and joint neuropathy, the weakness or numbness caused by nerve damage. A 2019 report published in the same journal concluded that CBD was effective enough in animal studies to warrant clinical trials in people.[74]

In a similar vein, a 2020 study by researchers at the University of New Mexico, Albuquerque, reported for the first time that full-spectrum hemp-extracted oil with negligible THC levels significantly improved pain levels in mice with chronic neuropathy-related pain.[75]

Finally, though human research is lagging, many people report arthritis pain relief from CBD. In fact, when the Arthritis Foundation surveyed 2,600 people with the disease (52 percent had osteoarthritis; 45 percent had rheumatoid arthritis), they found that 79 percent were using CBD to treat their symptoms.[76]

Participants in the 2019 Project CBD survey also gave the supplement two thumbs up for pain management. Just shy of 90 percent of participants said they experienced some improvement in the frequency and duration of their pain, with 60 percent reporting that CBD made these aspects "much better." Even more significant was CBD's impact on their perception of pain intensity: Before taking CBD, the average pain score was 6.85; when taking CBD, the average pain score was just 2.76—a 60 percent decrease in their pain's intensity.[77]

The Arthritis Foundation suggests starting with low doses (e.g., 5 mg to 10 mg twice a day) and increasing if you feel no relief. You can also use CBD topically as well as orally, depending on the type of pain you have. Always let your doctor know what supplements, including CBD, you are taking, especially if you're already taking medications for pain or other conditions.[78]

COVID-19

A S THE COVID-19 pandemic brought the world to a halt, some unscrupulous and overzealous CBD proponents started pushing CBD oil as an antiviral cure-all. It's not. The CBD picture is complicated when it comes to viral immunity, especially COVID-19 immunity and one of its more severe complications, the cytokine storm syndrome.

> There is no evidence that cannabinoids protect against or increase the risk of infection.

Characterized by intense immune overreaction in the lungs, this little understood syndrome can sicken and kill infected individuals. Respiratory distress is the leading cause of mortality in COVID-19 cases. The critically ill who survive intensive care may suffer long-term lung and/ or neurological damage, resulting in functional impairment and reduced quality of life.

Science Daily reported that a hyperinflammatory cytokine storm, involving a surge of immune cells gone haywire, was likely the primary cause of death in several viral outbreaks, including the 1918–20 "Spanish flu" pandemic (which killed more than 50 million people) and, more recently, the H1N1 swine flu and the so-called bird flu.

In cases of viral-induced acute pulmonary distress, anti-cytokine-storm targeted therapy would seem to make sense. In hyperinflammation, immunosuppression can be beneficial. But treatment with anti-inflammatory corticosteroids is not a great option because it can exacerbate COVID-19-associated lung injury.

Could anti-inflammatory cannabinoids like CBD and THC calm a cytokine storm? In theory, it would seem plausible. Medical scientists in Israel have launched a study to assess CBD's potential as a treatment for a COVID-induced cytokine storm, but it's far too early to draw conclusions. The interplay between cannabinoids and the

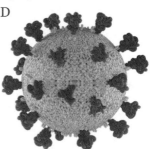

immune system is complex and in some ways paradoxical—sometimes CBD and THC suppress immunity and sometimes they appear to boost immune function.

The best way to look at it is that cannabinoids can modulate immune activity in both directions. They keep inflammation in check under healthy conditions but enable an inflammatory response when needed to fight infection. Mariano García de Palau, MD, a Spanish clinician, sums it up this way: "I believe [cannabis] is immunosuppressive when there is a hyper-immune response, but otherwise it regulates and corrects the immune system. In fact, you could say it functions like the endocannabinoid system, bringing equilibrium to the organism." [79]

What does this mean, practically speaking, for those who are choosing to use CBD during the COVID-19 pandemic? Will consuming small amounts of CBD as a preventive measure help to strengthen our immune resistance? Or could it make us more susceptible to the coronavirus by suppressing our immunity? Only a relatively small percentage of people with COVID-19 experience a life-threatening cytokine storm, but if one is infected (without showing severe symptoms) would CBD mitigate or increase the risk of serious disease progression? Would CBD have any impact at all?

The International Association for Cannabinoid Medicine (IACM), based in Germany, issued a statement on the COVID-19 pandemic and the use of cannabinoids, noting that some laboratory studies suggest that cannabinoids may have antiviral effects. Thus far, however, according to the IACM, "There is no evidence that individual cannabinoids—such as CBD, CBG or THC—or cannabis preparations protect against infection... or could be used to treat COVID-19, the disease produced by this virus." But the IACM also emphasizes "there is no evidence that the use of cannabinoids could increase the risk of viral infection."

Even if CBD isn't especially useful in the ongoing battle with COVID-19, it most definitely can help combat the anxiety and depression that accompany prolonged stress and isolation. Rodent research shows that stress caused by being restrained causes a significant drop in anandamide in the corticolimbic brain regions, which are involved with emotion regulation, and eventually leads to a state of depression.[80] In that respect, CBD may be helpful for those who feel anxious and constrained while social distancing and remaining under quarantine during the extraordinarily stressful COVID-19 pandemic.

Dementia and Alzheimer's

ABOUT HALF OF older adults worry about developing memory loss and dementia, according to a University of Michigan's National Poll on Healthy Aging. Three quarters of the more than 1,000 surveyed adults try to strengthen their mental acuity and fend off mental deterioration by playing brain-training games and puzzles and by taking vitamins and other supplements.[81] Increasingly, research suggests that CBD should be among those other supplements.[82]

According to Dementia Care Central—a consumer education program developed with funding from the National Institute on Aging—the dementia-related conditions that can be helped by CBD include:
- Alzheimer's disease
- vascular dementia
- dementia with Lewy bodies (DLB)
- Parkinson's disease
- frontotemporal dementia
- Huntington's disease[83]

As is the case with CBD in general, the research done so far has largely been on animals and on cells in the laboratory. Human trials are needed before we know the real benefit of CBD against these devastating diseases, but the preliminary evidence is promising.

Cannabinoids "protect neurons on the molecular level," concluded a report in the *Philosophical Transactions of the Royal Society,* a British science journal. "Neuroinflammatory processes contributing to the progression of normal brain ageing and to the pathogenesis of neurodegenerative diseases are suppressed by cannabinoids."[84]

CBD is not only neuroprotective, it facilitates neurogenesis, the creation of new brain cells, which prevents mental deterioration and promotes brain health. And CBD reduces inflammation in the brain[85] and helps relax and open blood vessels for improved circulation and lower blood pressure.[86]

CBD also promotes brain health by reducing what is known as *glutamate excitotoxicity,* which can occur with stroke, brain trauma, and neurodegenerative disease like Alzheimer's.[87, 88] Too much excitation can damage or destroy a cell. Glutamate is the brain's main excitatory neurotransmitter. Our endogenous cannabinoid levels rise after a head injury or stroke-induced surge of glutamate. Similarly, plant cannabinoids like CBD and THC can help to protect the brain by countering an excess of glutamate.

A 2017 study published in *Frontiers in Pharmacology* reported that CBD reverses and prevents the development of cognitive deficits in animal models of Alzheimer's disease studies and that it may work even better when combined with THC. The researchers concluded, "The studies provide 'proof of principle' that CBD and possibly CBD-THC combinations are valid candidates for novel AD [Alzheimer's disease] therapies."[89]

This supports a growing body of evidence that cannabis may help fend off Alzheimer's disease. A 2016 study from the Salk Institute reported that THC and other compounds found in marijuana can promote the cellular removal of amyloid beta, proteins that clump together between neurons and form the plaques that are the hallmarks of Alzheimer's disease.

"Although other studies have offered evidence that cannabinoids might be neuroprotective against the symptoms of Alzheimer's, we believe our study is the first to demonstrate that cannabinoids affect both inflammation and amyloid beta accumulation in nerve cells," said Salk professor David Schubert, PhD, the senior author of the paper.[90]

Depression

DEPRESSION IS A serious condition that can lead to a variety of emotional and physical problems and hinder your ability to function. Symptoms include:
- fatigue
- anxiety
- irritability
- restlessness
- loss of enjoyment
- appetite changes
- changes in sleep patterns
- thoughts of death or suicide

Endocannabinoid system activity in the brain affects your moods and emotions, including feelings of anxiety and depression.[91] Pioneering neurologist and endocannabinoid researcher Ethan Russo, MD, suggested that depression might be a product of endocannabinoid deficiency, meaning low levels of these important mood regulators could lead to depression.[92] Scientific studies support this theory. In a 2008 study of women who had been diagnosed with depression, researchers reported that 2-AG levels were significantly decreased in the women with major depression; the longer the women were depressed, the lower their 2-AG levels.[93]

Also, when pharmaceutical companies released the obesity drug rimonabant, which was designed to block CB_1 receptors and reduce appetite, they ended up quickly pulling it off the market because of serious psychiatric side effects such as depression, anxiety, and suicidal thoughts.

The connection between the ECS and mood is undeniable. Supporting the endocannabinoid system is one way that CBD may help alleviate or prevent depression. CBD is also neuroprotective, and it promotes the development of new brain cells, specifically in the hippocampus, a process that has an antidepressant effect. Remember, too, that CBD helps manage stress and inflammation, which also wreak havoc on the body and can increase risk for depression.

Anecdotally, many people using CBD report positive results for depression. In Project CBD's 2019 survey, almost 90 percent of participants using CBD for a mood disorder reported that they had anxiety, which for most went hand-in-hand with depression. CBD significantly improved both anxiety and depression, according to the survey results.[94]

As with most conditions, we need more clinical research on how CBD affects people who are depressed.

Diabetes

DIABETES IS A condition in which your body does not properly process sugar. It can cause nerve damage, eye problems, heart disease, and stroke. Symptoms include:
- fatigue
- blurred vision
- feelings of thirst
- slow healing of cuts and bruises
- neuropathy, a nerve disorder that causes tingling, pain, or numbness in the hands and feet

Eating a diet high in sugar and refined carbohydrates sends our CB$_1$ receptors into overdrive and disrupts ECS tone, leading to poor appetite regulation and weight gain, which paves the way for metabolic disease. So it is not surprising that diets heavy in these foods are also linked to diabetes.

> CBD lowered the incidence of diabetes in laboratory rats.

We also know that the endocannabinoid system plays an integral role in regulating glucose metabolism and insulin sensitivity (how well our bodies process blood sugar) and that insulin resistance and high blood sugar leads to diabetes. So it makes sense that using CBD to enhance ESC tone could be helpful in the treatment and/or prevention of this common metabolic disease. Preliminary research is promising. A 2006 Israeli study found that CBD lowered the incidence of diabetes in laboratory rats, and human studies are currently underway.[95, 96]

CBD's anti-inflammatory properties also help keep insulin resistance in check. As diabetes develops, the body becomes less sensitive to insulin. That insulin resistance triggers inflammation, which can set up a vicious cycle with more inflammation leading to increasing insulin resistance and so on. CBD may help break the cycle.[97]

Helping to control chronic stress is another way CBD may help lessen the risk for diabetes. Research finds that high levels of stress over time can cause high levels of cortisol, which encourages fat storage, leads to high blood sugar, and increases the risk of developing type 2 diabetes.[98]

CBD may also help with weight loss, which can lower the risk for type 2 diabetes and reverse the condition in people who have it. That's particularly true for people who have excess abdominal fat, the hallmark of metabolic syndrome, a condition linked to type 2 diabetes. Your belly fat is like an independent organ all its own, disrupting your normal, healthy hormone balance and increasing your risk for insulin resistance and diabetes.

Finally, there is anecdotal evidence from people living with diabetes that CBD can help control the condition. In the 2019 Project CBD survey, participants taking CBD for diabetes were asked their average blood sugar levels before and after they started taking CBD. Though average blood sugar levels with CBD were still high, they showed significant improvements over the pre-CBD levels, decreasing from 178 to 130 on average. Participants also reported significant improvements in neuropathy-type symptoms (i.e., nerve pain, tingling, or numbness) and some improvements in their ability to maintain a healthy weight.

It's important to work with your doctor before taking CBD for diabetes, especially if you manage your diabetes with medication. CBD might interfere with some of the blood sugar–lowering effects of common diabetes drugs like Metformin.[99]

Digestive and Bowel Disorders

DIGESTIVE AND BOWEL disorders include inflammatory bowel disease (IBD) such as ulcerative colitis and Crohn's disease, as well as irritable bowel syndrome (IBS).

IBD and IBS sound similar and are often (mistakenly) used interchangeably, but they are different conditions. IBS is not actually a disease but rather a group of symptoms that include abdominal pain, cramping, diarrhea and/or constipation. In IBS, which is sometimes referred to as "spastic colon," the colon (also known as the bowel or large intestine) is not working properly, moving either too slowly or too quickly. Doctors generally recommend changes in diet and stress management to help alleviate it.

IBD is an umbrella term to describe a variety of diseases, including Crohn's disease and ulcerative colitis, which are the two main types of IBD, as well as pouchitis and microscopic colitis. Crohn's disease can affect any part of the GI tract but typically causes inflammatory damage to the small intestine and the start of the colon. Ulcerative colitis causes inflammation of the colon and rectum. Symptoms can be digestive, such as diarrhea, bloody stools, abdominal pain, cramping, nausea, and constipation as well as more systemic symptoms, such as fatigue, fever, and joint pain.

CBD may be helpful for both IBS and IBD, but in different ways. IBS is one of the diseases that renowned cannabinoid researcher Dr. Ethan Russo categorized as a condition associated with clinical endocannabinoid deficiency. Considering that the GI tract is rich in CB receptors and the endocannabinoid system regulates digestive behavior, it makes sense that supporting the ECS with cannabinoids like CBD could provide relief. Inflammation is at the root of IBD, and CBD is known to be a potent anti-inflammatory, so it appears to be a natural, gentle fit to help alleviate these types of diseases.[100]

That said, hard scientific evidence supporting CBD for IBD is relatively sparse, though there are a handful of studies that show promise for reducing the worst of the symptoms. One 2018 Israeli study of 46 people with moderately severe Crohn's disease reported that CBD-rich cannabis oil (which also contained 4 percent THC) significantly improved symptoms, including diarrhea and abdominal pain, in 65 percent of the volunteers after eight weeks. Interestingly, though, endoscopic tests on the participants revealed that the treatment didn't actually reduce the inflammation in their guts, so how it worked is unclear.[101, 102]

"We know that cannabinoids can have profound anti-inflammatory effects, but this study indicates that the improvement in symptoms may not be related to these anti-inflammatory properties," the lead author, Timna Naftali, MD, reported.

A study by British doctors (supported by British pharmaceutical company GW

CBD May Build a Healthy Biome

Your gut microbiome is comprised of trillions of bacteria and other microbes. This enormous colony does far more than help you digest the food you eat, though it certainly does that. It helps regulate the immune system; produces essential nutrients, including vitamins B12, riboflavin, and vitamin K; and plays an instrumental role in keeping us healthy.

When the microbiome is dysfunctional, we experience gut dysbiosis and become more susceptible to illness of all kinds, including autoimmune diseases, obesity, diabetes, Parkinson's, and heart disease. The microbiome even affects our moods and behaviors through a channel known as the gut-brain axis.

The endocannabinoid system regulates your gut-brain axis, facilitating communication between the gut biome and the brain. Gut dysbiosis sends an unhealthy message to the brain that makes one more susceptible to overeating and metabolic imbalance. University of California

scientists in Riverside reported that dysregulated gut-brain signaling drives overeating associated with obesity.[103]

"Although the exact mechanisms are not well understood, evidence is mounting to support the role of probiotic intervention in reducing anxiety and stress response," Italian researchers reported in a 2013 study published in the *Journal of Pediatric Gastroenterology and Nutrition*.[104]

The best way to maintain a healthy, diverse gut biome is by eating a wide variety of probiotic foods like yogurt, kefir, sauerkraut, pickles, kombucha, tempeh, and pickles, which contain beneficial bacteria, and prebiotic foods like artichoke, garlic, onions, leeks, asparagus, and green bananas, which feed your gut bacteria.[105] Certain herbs and spices also have a positive impact on the gut microbiome.

Recent research has shown that THC is a probiotic compound that stimulates the growth of beneficial bacteria. According to ECS researcher Dr. Ethan Russo, "THC

actually stimulates production of some of the more beneficial bacterium and suppresses the disease-causing bacteria."[106]

Animal studies demonstrate that the probiotic benefits of THC can prevent weight gain caused by eating a high-fat diet, possibly because of positive changes to the gut microbiome that maintain metabolic balance and discourage the formation of fat cells. It's worth noting that a study of nearly 8,500 adults found that current cannabis users were much less likely to develop metabolic syndrome (which raises your risk for obesity and other diseases) than nonusers.[107]

Although it is not known to provide the same probiotic benefits as THC, CBD can support a healthy microbiome by toning the endocannabinoid system, which regulates communication via the gut-brain axis. Just remember, CBD doesn't replace the need for a healthy, gut biome–building diet. CBD augments a good diet, and a good diet enhances the health-

Pharmaceuticals) echoed these findings. This time the researchers tested CBD-rich extract on people with ulcerative colitis. Volunteers took capsules containing 50 mg of CBD and an "appreciable amount" of THC at a dose of 300 mg to 500 mg of CBD (up to 10 capsules) a day. They reported some relief from their ulcerative colitis symptoms, such as cramping, pain, and diarrhea and improvements in quality of life with CBD treatment, though again the treatment didn't appear to have appreciable benefits on reducing the inflammation itself.[108, 109]

Finally, in 2019, medical researchers based in Ohio examined the medical records of people with Crohn's disease to determine the prevalence of disease complications among cannabis users versus complications among nonusers.[110] Cannabis users reported 40 to 70 percent fewer symptoms. Two thirds as many cannabis users as nonusers (11.5 percent vs. 15.9 percent) had active complications like abdominal abscesses. And cannabis users were almost three times less likely to require treatment with TPN, an intravenous nutrient. According to the authors, "Our study suggests that cannabis use may mitigate several of the well-described complications of Crohn's disease among hospital inpatients."[111]

In the case of IBS, CBD may provide relief by toning the endocannabinoid system, which helps regulate the GI tract and the gut-brain connection. A 2020 study published in *Frontiers in Neuroscience* suggested that manipulating the ECS could be considered a primary target for managing IBS, concluding: "Although the pathophysiology of IBS remains unclear, targeting the ECS may represent a promising strategy...that may improve IBS symptoms onset."[112]

Stress can aggravate the gut, so gastroenterologists often recommend stress-reduction strategies as one of the ways to relieve

> CBD may provide relief by toning the endocannabinoid system.

symptoms of IBS. CBD is known to help assuage stress, which may be another way the cannabinoid helps with IBS.

In Project CBD's 2019 survey, among people taking CBD for GI diseases, particularly IBS, CBD appears to be very helpful for relieving abdominal cramps and pain, nausea, vomiting, and indigestion. Many respondents reported that it helped with their fatigue, though some found it made them more tired (perhaps because they were using a large dose or the product contained other ingredients that had a sedating effect). CBD did not appear to help people with GI diseases maintain a healthy weight; half of participants in this group reported either no change or a worsening of the weight gain and/or loss (it can cause either) that's often a problem with IBS.

Epilepsy

EPILEPSY IS A central nervous system (neurological) disorder in which your brain's circuitry and activity become abnormal, causing seizures or periods of unusual behavior, sensations, and sometimes loss of awareness. Symptoms of a seizure can include temporary confusion, a staring spell, uncontrolled jerking of arms and legs, loss of consciousness, and sudden rapid eye movement. Seizures are a symptom of epilepsy, but not all people who have seizures have epilepsy. About 1 in every 100 people will have an unprovoked seizure in their lifetime. About 4 percent of people will develop epilepsy in their life.[113]

In summer 2018, the FDA approved the first (and currently only) CBD-based drug called Epidiolex, produced by GW Pharmaceuticals, a British company. Extensive clinical trials showed that Epidiolex (a nearly pure CBD drug) can reduce severe, otherwise untreatable seizures in children who have two rare forms of epilepsy, Dravet syndrome and Lennox-Gestaut syndrome. Two years later, the FDA indicated that Epidiolex could also be used to treat seizures in patients with a genetic disorder called tuberous sclerosis complex.

Though it feels new and revolutionary, the U.S. Pharmacopeia

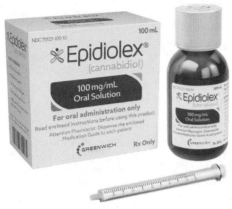

Epidiolex

listed cannabis tincture as a treatment for seizures and childhood convulsions back in the mid-1800s. Forty years ago, scientists first noted that CBD; in particular, shows promise as an antiepileptic remedy. In a study published in 1980, researchers gave eight volunteers with epilepsy a daily dose of 200 mg to 300 mg of CBD for four and a half months to see if they could alleviate their symptoms. Half of them saw dramatic improvements and remained almost free from convulsive attacks throughout the study period; three of the volunteers experienced partial improvement, and only one of the study participants experienced no improvement.[114, 115]

But there was little immediate follow-up on these tantalizing results until medical cannabis patients in California and Colorado, left to their own devices, discovered the profound antiseizure properties of CBD-rich cannabis oil. Stories about CBD's seemingly miraculous curative powers for epileptic children were broadcast on national television in 2013, setting the stage for FDA approval of pharmaceutical CBD five years later.

Epidiolex is a big step forward for CBD acceptance in the medical community. However, CBD-rich whole-plant extracts, which contain other cannabinoids and cannabis compounds, may be better medicine than a CBD isolate product that contains additives like ethanol and sucralose, found in Epidiolex.

In a 2018 meta-analysis study, Brazilian scientists examined 11 different studies comprising 670 people who took CBD for their epilepsy

"I Tried It"

Sadie Higuera, 7,
Ramona, California

SADIE HIGUERA was born with a rare genetic condition called Schinzel-Giedion syndrome, which made her chances of survival low and frequency of seizures quite extreme. Experiencing nearly 300 life-threatening seizures each day, little Sadie rarely saw relief from them. But when her parents began treating her with CBD oil, they immediately saw results. Sadie's eyes were focusing, and her seizures subsided. "CBD has improved our family's quality of life in every way possible," said Brian Higuera, Sadie's father.

Today, 7-year-old Sadie takes both CBD oil and cannabis oil with THC. She is almost seizure-free, makes sounds, and is sitting up on her own. "Sadie wasn't even able to have occupational or physical therapy prior to taking CBD oil since her doctor didn't think the return would be worth the time and resources," Higuera said. Now she "goes to school and comes on family vacations—all of which we never thought was possible before."

Additionally, Sadie is no longer on the plethora of medications that were originally prescribed to her. Thanks to the oil, she no longer has to take them. "When we first started giving Sadie CBD oil, she was on 14 different medications," Higuera said. "Now, she isn't on any. She takes iron supplements and additional supplements but is not on any prescribed medications."

for an average of six months. The researchers found that 71 percent of people using CBD-rich extracts had reduced seizure frequency, compared with 46 percent of those using Epidiolex. What's more, the participants in this analysis had a history of being resistant to treatment and had tried between 4 and 12 medications for three years before using CBD.[116]

The researchers also examined how many of the participants had greater than 50 percent reduction of seizures (a typical threshold used in medicine) as well as how many had a greater than 70 percent improvement. Both the whole-plant extracts and CBD isolates helped reduce the number of seizures in half for roughly 40 percent of the participants. Both formulations reduced seizures by 70 percent in about one quarter of the study volunteers, but fewer studies reported this. And roughly 1 in 10 of the participants using CBD became seizure-free, although not enough studies reported this result to compare different formulations. So both the isolate and whole-plant product worked, but one striking difference was the dosages.

The average dosage for people using pure CBD was 25.3 mg/kg/day, but for CBD-rich extracts it was 6.0 mg/kg/day. In other words, CBD in a whole-plant extract was over four times more potent than isolated CBD, likely due to the benefits of the entourage effect.

People taking whole-plant CBD also had fewer side effects. High doses of Epidiolex were associated with mild adverse side effects, such as fatigue, nausea, and GI problems in 73 percent of people taking it, whereas whole-plant CBD was associated with these types of side effects in only 33 percent of cases. The difference may be due to the lower dose of CBD used when formulated as a whole-plant extract, as well as the fact that Epidiolex includes additives like ethanol and sucralose, which may contribute to unwanted side effects.[117]

Fibromyalgia and Chronic Fatigue Syndrome

F IBROMYALGIA IS A difficult-to-treat condition defined by chronic, widespread pain and debilitation. It is also one of the conditions that Dr. Ethan Russo hypothesized may be the result of clinical endocannabinoid deficiency syndrome, in which the body isn't making enough of its own endogenous cannabinoids to properly regulate the many physiological systems under its control. If that's the case, then taking plant cannabinoids like CBD and THC could address the root of the disease rather than merely mitigating some symptoms.

Current research supports that theory. In a 2020 study published in *Clinical and Experimental Rheumatology*, Italian researchers demonstrated that cannabis can be used effectively to remedy fibromyalgia symptoms, at least by some patients.[118]

The researchers recruited fibromyalgia patients at the Luigi Sacco

University Hospital in Milan, Italy. Sixty-six of them were interviewed over six months of treatment. The average participant was 52 years old, and over 90 percent of sufferers were women (women make up the vast majority of people with fibromyalgia).

The study focused on treating refractory patients—people who are taking and tolerating medications but haven't found relief. Just under half of the participants were taking two other drugs, while nearly a third were taking at least three. These drugs were strong central nervous system sedatives, including opioids, anticonvulsants, nerve blockers, and antidepressants.

"I Tried It"

Melinda Misuraca, 57, Figueiro dos Vinhos, Portugal

IN A PERSONAL ESSAY published by Project CBD, Melinda Misuraca (who developed the recipes in this book) described how her once-dependable good health suddenly failed her. From room-spinning vertigo to mysterious rashes, excruciating pain to constant nausea, her symptoms soon overwhelmed her.

"I felt as though I was being swallowed alive, my life force squeezed out of me," she says. "In a few weeks' time, I had morphed from a high-functioning writer, professor, and parent into a sobbing lump of misery who could no longer drive a car, read a book, wash a dish, or hold a pen. I was so weak that a routine task—like taking a shower—would flatten me for hours."

After tests, scans, and visits with multiple doctors, she finally had a diagnosis: myalgic encephalomyelitis (ME), also known as chronic fatigue syndrome (CFS).

According to the Centers for Disease Control and Prevention (CDC), about 2.5 million people in the United States and 17 million worldwide suffer from ME/CFS, which renders 75 percent of sufferers disabled, with 25 percent homebound and even bedridden.

"Chronic fatigue syndrome is a very challenging disease," says Robert K. Naviaux, MD, head of the Mitochondrial and Metabolic Disease Center at UC San Diego School of Medicine. "It affects multiple systems of the body. Symptoms vary and are common to many other diseases. There is no diagnostic laboratory test." There are no FDA-approved treatments, and any medications doctors prescribe are off-label and fraught with adverse side effects.

Misuraca tried medica-

The participants were given two formulations: one was THC rich and the other was balanced with a bit more CBD than THC. They used the balanced formula early in the day and the THC-rich formula in the evening.

Nearly half of participants (47 percent) got enough relief from these cannabis formulations to reduce or cease their painkiller usage. Between a third and half of the participants experienced improvements in sleep, anxiety, depression, and pain symptoms. The majority of participants were overweight or obese, and cannabis seemed to be more effective for heavier patients.

tions for pain, sleep, and depression, but nothing helped. Forced to quit the teaching job she loved, she drained her dwindling funds on all kinds of alternative therapies. She gave up gluten, sugar, and animal products. She tried supplements, massage, and acupuncture. Then she heard that some people with ME/CFS found cannabis to be helpful. "I hadn't smoked weed in years," said Misuraca, "and, frankly, getting stoned sounded like the last thing a completely incapacitated person ought to do. But I was willing to try anything."

A resident of California at the time, she obtained a recommendation for medical marijuana and went to a dispensary. After taking her first hit of a THC-rich joint that night, she said, "The background noise of paralyzing pain grew quiet, and a calming sensation washed over me. I effortlessly floated off to sleep for the first time in more than a year. In the morning I felt different—not cured, but hopeful."

When she added CBD to her cannabis regimen, more symptoms relinquished their stranglehold. "I began to read and write again. One night, I went to see my daughter's theater performance, the first evening I'd been out in a year. With the help of homegrown CBD-rich cannabis, I was coming back to life."

These days, Misuraca says, "I am functioning at about 80 percent of my physiological capacity—and that feels like remission to me. I manage my health by eating a mostly plant-based diet, exercise, stress reduction, some supplements, and daily dosing with a CBD-rich tincture, with occasional THC-rich cannabis at night. I won't claim that cannabis completely cured my ME/CFS, but I will say that, as part of a broader healing protocol, it has helped immensely. I hardly think about my diagnosis anymore. There are other mysteries I'm curious about, and I'm busy unraveling them, and in the meantime, I'm thriving."[119]

Regarding CBD itself, a study published in 2017 suggested that it may be able to turn down the activity of brain cells called *glia* that can lead to a condition known as *central sensitization,* where the entire nervous system becomes overly sensitive to everyday stimulation like bright light, noise, textures, strong odors, and temperature extremes, which may be the mechanism behind conditions like fibromyalgia and chronic fatigue.[120, 121]

In chronic fatigue syndrome (CFS), also known as myalgic encephalomyelitis (ME), the immune system, spurred by an unknown cause, goes into full aberrant fight mode, activating a hyperinflammatory response and setting off a nightmarish carnival of symptoms. A 2015 article in *Science Advances* reported heightened immune activity in people with ME/CFS during the early phase of the disease that was "consistent with a viral trigger or disrupted immune regulatory networks."[122] But in later stages, the levels of immune disturbance were much lower. It appears that whatever immunological threat initially triggered the disease could have been resolved—and yet the body continued its inflammatory, foe-fighting stance.

Given that a runaway immune response and marked inflammation are major players in ME/CFS, it makes sense that both CBD and THC, two potent anti-inflammatory compounds, could be profoundly therapeutic. Anecdotal evidence bears this out. As Melinda Misuraca, a Project CBD contributor and ME/CFS sufferer, wrote, "Inflammation and pain are like conjoined demon twins" that CBD and THC go a long way toward taming.

Heart Disease

HEART DISEASE IS a catchall phrase for the disease that develops when the arteries of the heart cannot deliver enough oxygen-rich blood to the heart, leading to events like heart attack. It's the leading cause of death in the United

States, killing about 655,000 Americans each year, which is about one in every four deaths.[123] Key risk factors for heart disease include unhealthy diet, physical inactivity, diabetes, overweight and obesity, and excessive alcohol use.

Similarly, a stroke, which is sometimes called " brain attack," occurs when blood flow to the brain is blocked or reduced. So the same precautions that protect against heart attacks and other cardiovascular disease (like diet, exercise, and a healthy lifestyle that can include CBD supplementation) can help prevent stroke. CBD can also play a key role in protecting the brain after a stroke. (For more on CBD's role in treating traumatic brain injury and stroke, see page 124.)

> CBD may also protect against cardiac arrhythmias, or irregular heartbeats.

Research shows that CBD can help maintain healthy cardiovascular function and prevent heart disease on a number of fronts, including protecting against hardening of the arteries, lowering blood pressure, and reducing the incidence of potentially dangerous arrhythmias.

It starts inside your arteries. When the linings of your artery walls are injured, they build up plaque that can cause the arteries to narrow. This is called *atherosclerosis*; it's a prevalent form of heart disease. Inflammation is a leading cause of this type of injury, as is high blood pressure. Exposure to tiny chronic doses of THC has been shown to slow the progression of atherosclerosis in animal studies.[124]

THC and CBD are both vasodilators, meaning they widen your blood vessels, a process regulated by the ECS. This can have a pronounced positive effect on blood pressure. In a 2017 study, British researchers gave a group of men either 600 mg of CBD or a dummy supplement and monitored their blood pressure at rest and again after stress tests that normally increased blood pressure. Just that single dose of CBD reduced the participants' resting systolic blood

"I Tried It"

Selene Yeager, 51,
Lehigh Valley,
Pennsylvania

FOR MOST OF HER ADULT LIFE, Selene Yeager, a 51-year-old coach, endurance athlete, and health and fitness writer (and the writer of this book!) didn't worry much about her blood pressure, which had generally hovered in the normal 120/80 range. But as she reached her late forties and entered perimenopause, she found those numbers creeping up. At one routine checkup, it was 138/80, a number she found concerning.

"My brother has high blood pressure despite being fit and active, and my parents both had heart disease, so I knew I wasn't immune. I bought a home blood pressure monitor so I could keep an eye on it," she says.

About the same time, a friend who had launched his own CBD company asked if she wanted to try some products, explaining that, as an anti-inflammatory, CBD could help her recover more quickly from hard training sessions and bike races.

Yeager started using a 1,200 mg full-spectrum tincture, which delivered 2 mg CBD per drop. Not knowing how it would affect her, she decided to take one serving—a dropperful containing 40 mg—before bed.

"I was pretty skeptical and didn't expect much. As a health and fitness writer and athlete, I've tried *a lot* of supplements and haven't been impressed with most of them," Yeager says. "Honestly, I didn't really notice that it helped me recover any faster after a

pressure by 6 mmHg. Plus, they had less of a spike in blood pressure in response to stress than those taking a single dose of a placebo pill.

In a follow-up study, where the researchers gave 26 men 600 mg of CBD or a placebo for seven days, the results were mixed.[125] Measurements of resting blood pressure revealed that the participants had developed a tolerance to the CBD over time, but CBD's ability to lower blood pressure during stress persisted. (Of course, if you are already dealing with low blood pressure, the blood pressure–reducing effects of CBD are something to be aware of, and you may need to avoid high doses.)[126]

"The reduction of arterial stiffness, and improvements in internal carotid artery blood flow and endothelial function after chronic CBD treatment, indicate a positive effect in vascular function that race or tough ride."

What she did notice was that it was helping her sleep better. "For years, I would wake up around 3 a.m. with my head full of racing thoughts and have trouble falling back asleep. When I started using a dropperful of the tincture before bed, I started sleeping straight through the night more often."

Her night sweats, something she had dealt with most of her adult life, which had gotten more frequent and severe as she entered perimenopause, also got better. "I wasn't waking up in a pool of sweat anymore,"

she says. She also noticed that she felt less anxious when working on stressful deadlines.

After a couple of months, she noticed something else: Her blood pressure had dipped to levels she'd never seen. "I had been traveling a lot and gotten out of the habit of checking it regularly. But one day I looked over in the corner of my home office and saw the blood pressure machine sitting there on top of a stack of books and thought, 'I should get back to checking that.' I put it on and sort of braced myself, a little worried it would be high."

It was 117/78. "I thought maybe I'd done something wrong, so I waited a couple of minutes and took it again. Similar number. I even replaced the battery in the machine and tested it again just to be sure!" she says.

Now it routinely hovers around 110/70, which Yeager attributes to the CBD. "I later learned that CBD is good for lowering blood pressure, and of course I was sleeping better and feeling lower levels of anxiety, which I'm sure also help," she says. "I've been taking it faithfully ever since."

warrants further investigation in relevant patient populations," lead researcher Saoirse E. O'Sullivan, PhD, reported.[127]

CBD may also protect against cardiac arrhythmias, or irregular heartbeats, where the heart beats too fast, too slowly, or with an irregular pattern. Arrhythmias can be brought on by long-term stress, as high cortisol levels can raise blood pressure, blood cholesterol, blood sugar, triglycerides, and other risk factors for heart disease in general. CBD's antianxiety properties can help combat stress, lower cortisol, and protect against arrhythmias related to those causes.

Research shows that CBD also can suppress irregular heartbeat caused by stroke-induced ischemia (inadequate blood supply to the heart) and can minimize tissue damage caused by the lack of oxygen.[128] A study published in the *British Journal of Pharmacology* found that when rats were given CBD 10 minutes before a 30-minute coronary artery occlusion (partial or complete obstruction of blood flow in the coronary artery, which may cause chest pain, heart attack, and tissue damage) or 10 minutes before blood flow was restored, they experienced fewer arrhythmias and less tissue damage than rats not given CBD. Research in this area is still in the early stage, but it already shows great potential.

Since cannabinoids also mop up free radicals—and improve the effects of other antioxidants in the body—CBD may also protect against heart disease by reducing the cellular damage that happens when we're exposed to free-radical producers like processed foods and environmental pollution.

CBD also delays the reabsorption of a chemical called adenosine (meaning that you have more of it in circulation), which quells inflammation and helps maintain healthy heart function.

If you're already taking medications for blood pressure, cholesterol, or other heart conditions, it's important to consult with your doctor before you start taking CBD. High doses of CBD may interfere with the metabolism of some of these drugs, which could have problematic consequences.[129]

Liver and Kidney Disease

CHRONIC LIVER DISEASE is a major public health problem affecting hundreds of millions of people throughout the world. Fatty liver, kidney disease, diabetes, and other diet-related metabolic disorders are expressions of overactive CB_1 receptor signaling and inadequate CB_2 receptor stimulation. CBD fine-tunes the ECS by turning down the CB_1 dimmer switch while mimicking and augmenting CB_2 activity.

In both the liver and kidneys (and other) internal organs, the CB_1 and CB_2 receptors have a yin-yang type of relationship. When the CB_1 receptor is overstimulated and there's not enough CB_2 receptor signaling—or vice versa—various diseases follow.[130]

In the liver and kidneys specifically, CB_1 signaling is profibrotic, meaning it encourages the development of fibrous connective tissue in response to injury or damage. CB_2 signaling is antifibrotic, meaning it impedes fibrosis and thins the blood. When CB_1 and CB_2 are out of balance, it can lead to fibrosis, or dangerous scarring on these organs. Cirrhosis of the liver and nonalcoholic liver disease are two serious conditions that are marked by too much fibrosis, which is also a characteristic of chronic kidney disease. Effective treatment strategies for fibrotic conditions should aim to boost CB_2 signaling, while fine-tuning CB_1 in the other direction. That's what CBD does, and that's how CBD may help to fend off disease and keep your liver and kidneys healthy.[131, 132]

CBD's ability to protect the liver was the focus of a 2017 study published in the journal *Scientific Reports*, which examined the effect of CBD on mice that had been given enough ethanol to mimic chronic and binge alcohol use. The study found that CBD oil minimized fat accumulation and damage to the liver.[133] The authors concluded: "CBD may have therapeutic potential in the treatment of alcoholic liver diseases associated with inflammation, oxidative stress and steatosis [fatty change], which deserves exploration in human trials."

In another study that examined the impact of CBD on liver health in animals, researchers gave lab rats CBD and other cannabinoids for eight months. Published in *Cell Death and Disease*, the study found that CBD killed off hepatic stellate cells (HSC), which trigger scar tissue in the liver.[134] "Not only does there not seem to be any evidence that CBD plays a role in damaging the liver over a long period of time," the scientists reported, "it actually seems that the cannabinoid may help to improve liver health and reduce the effects of any damage done to it. More studies continue to be required, particularly those involving human participants. However, current evidence appears to support the notion that CBD oil use is not only safe, but it may even have a potentially therapeutic role in treating liver disease."[135]

This assessment calls into question the FDA's warnings, based on weak evidence, that CBD may harm the liver. We'll take a closer look at those warnings in Chapter 10.

Migraine and Headache Disorders

MIGRAINE IS A recurrent throbbing headache that typically affects one side of your head and is often accompanied by nausea and disturbed vision. Sufferers may also experience sensitivity to light, sound, smell, or touch; nausea and vomiting; light-headedness; and blurred vision. About 12 percent of people experience migraines. It's more common in women than men.[136]

Migraine is also one of the conditions that neurologist Dr. Ethan Russo categorized as a clinical endocannabinoid deficiency disorder. People who suffer from migraines are thought to have low levels of anandamide, he says, so "normal sensations in the brain are magnified to the point of becoming painful when they would not be to a person free from the affliction."[137]

If cannabinoid deficiency is at the root of these monster headaches, it makes sense that balancing the endocannabinoid system could be beneficial. There's also historical precedence for using cannabinoids for migraines. Prominent physicians from the mid-1800s to the mid-1900s were prescribing cannabis oil tinctures to treat migraines.[138] Current research also supports medical marijuana for migraine prevention and pain relief.

A 2017 study presented at the Congress of the European Academy of Neurology concluded that "cannabinoids are suitable for migraine

"I Tried It"

VJ Von Art, 37,
London, United Kingdom

A S A SUFFERER of chronic fatigue syndrome/myalgic encephalomyelitis, VJ Von Art developed crippling insomnia that also triggered anxiety and migraines. "The migraines were so intense that most of the time I had to go to the hospital to treat them," Von Art said. "I was running out of options." Then, one day she decided to try CBD—and for her, it changed everything.

"The first week I took CBD before going to bed, it felt as if an external force had overwritten my mental chatter and my brain went to sleep within 5 to 10 minutes," Von Art said. "CBD gave me the well-needed rest and lifted the mental fog I had from chronic fatigue syndrome."

CBD helped reduce both the frequency and severity of her migraines. Before, she got them once a week and "it could explode into a three-day episode." Now, she only gets them only two to three times a year, which are relieved by over-the-counter painkillers. If the headache is severe, combining CBD with an OTC painkiller "boosts the effect of the medication and nips the pain in the bud pretty fast."

prophylaxis [preventing migraines]." In this study, 79 people who suffered from chronic migraines received a daily dose of either 25 mg amitriptyline (a tricyclic antidepressant often used to treat migraine) or 200 mg of a THC-CBD combination tincture for three months. Forty-eight people who suffered from cluster headaches—relatively short but extremely painful headaches that can keep recurring for days, weeks, or even months—received either 200 mg THC-CBD or a daily dose of 480 mg verapamil (a calcium blocker that prevents the constriction of blood vessels occurring prior to a migraine attack).[139] When volunteers experienced either type of headache, they took 200 mg of THC-CBD for acute pain relief.

After 12 to 16 weeks, both the amitriptyline and THC-CBD treatment groups had a 40 percent reduction in migraine headaches. Cannabinoids reduced pain intensity in migraine sufferers by 43.5 percent, yet the same results were only observed in cluster headache patients who had experienced migraine in childhood. Among cluster headache sufferers with no migraine history, THC-CBD had no effect.[140] Scientific evidence for CBD alone as a treatment for migraines is lacking, though it does appear to help with pain in general by increasing endocannabinoid levels in your brain and body.

A survey of 120 adults in Colorado who used cannabis to prevent migraines found that the users had half their usual migraine attacks, dropping from 10.4 to 4.6 per month. More than 85 percent of the group enjoyed fewer migraines.[141]

Though medical marijuana could reduce migraine frequency, there simply isn't enough evidence to say CBD alone (without THC) is effective against migraines and similar headaches. The American Migraine Foundation says that topical CBD salve could be useful to relieve the joint and muscle pain associated with migraine and that CBD oil (or better yet, some CBDA) might prevent nausea and vomiting often associated with migraine.

Nausea

I F YOU WERE to point to a single condition that helped push medical marijuana into the mainstream, it's nausea. Marijuana's efficacy for easing chemo-induced nausea for cancer patients and people with AIDS was a major impetus for the emergence of medical marijuana as a major social movement in the United States. There is no disputing that THC-rich cannabis helps nausea, and CBD is very effective against it as well.

It works so well that even those leery of trying anything cannabis-related are pleasantly surprised by how quickly they feel much better with the right dosage. Stacey Kerr, MD, a teacher, physician, and author living and working in Northern California, shared a story with Project CBD:

"Laura was a physician who spent much of her clinical time treating substance abuse disorders, [so her] aversion to using cannabis when she was going through chemotherapy for breast

cancer did not surprise me. Finally, I introduced her to a calibrated vaporizer—a method of administration that could provide quick relief but was different than the 'smoke a joint out behind the barn' approach she had imagined. She started with a CBD-rich herb and [I was thrilled when she] reported, 'It worked faster, better, and more completely than any of the prescriptions my oncologist gave me.'"[142]

> CBD has been shown to alleviate both nausea and vomiting.

In acute cases, like when you have an infection or food poisoning, nausea and vomiting serve as defense mechanisms to purge your body of offending invaders and make you well. Nausea can also be chronic, as in the case of pregnancy and the miserable side effects of chemotherapy, migraine, psychiatric disorders, and other conditions.

Nausea occurs when receptors in your brain, GI tract, and nervous system work together to trigger the gut to produce more serotonin,[143] which in high enough levels stimulates the nausea area of the brain as a protective mechanism.[144] Antiemetic (antivomiting) medications work by blocking the nauseating effects of serotonin release. CBD can work the same way.

CBD reacts with serotonin-releasing receptors and in relatively small doses has been shown to help alleviate both nausea and vomiting. It also helps ease anxiety, which can help people manage the emotional discomfort of chronic nausea, such as during chemotherapy.

THC also works against nausea by binding to CB_1 receptors in specific areas of the brain to reduce vomiting. In the right doses, the mood-elevating effects of THC also can create a more positive mind-set for people who are going through chemotherapy. That's important because the negative expectations of treatment can lead to anticipatory nausea, which is difficult to counteract with traditional meds.

Animal studies show that CBDA, the acidic, raw form of CBD (which converts to CBD over time and when heated), may be even more effective against nausea than either CBD or THC.[145, 146] While scientific research into CBDA and other cannabinoid acids proceeds at a slow pace, some medical cannabis dispensaries are offering CBDA products for people who need them. CBDA may also be found in some raw hemp oil (not hemp seed oil) products that have not been decarboxylated or heated in processing.

Parkinson's Disease

PARKINSON'S DISEASE IS the second most common neurological disorder (after Alzheimer's disease) and affects about one million Americans. Parkinson's disease is most associated with compromised motor function after the loss of 60 percent to 80 percent of dopamine-producing neurons. As these neurons become damaged or die and the brain is less able to produce adequate amounts of dopamine, people may experience:

- tremor of the hands, arms, legs, or jaw
- muscle rigidity or stiffness of the limbs and trunk
- slowness of movement (bradykinesia)
- impaired balance and coordination (postural instability)
- decreased facial expressions
- dementia or confusion
- fatigue
- sleep disturbances
- depression
- constipation
- cognitive changes
- fear
- anxiety
- urinary problems

Uncontrolled Parkinson's disease significantly reduces quality of life and can render a person unable to care for themselves, trapped in a body they cannot control.[147]

Within a brain affected by Parkinson's disease, there are an inordinate number of *Lewy bodies,* protein clusters that cause dysfunction and neuronal degeneration. These Lewy bodies, coupled with the demise of dopamine-producing neurons, are considered to be hallmarks of Parkinson's. But mounting evidence suggests that these aberrations are actually advanced-stage manifestations of a slowly evolving disease process, as Nishi Whitely, author of *Chronic Relief: A Guide to Cannabis for the Terminally & Chronically Ill,* reported for Project CBD.

It appears that non-motor symptoms such as constipation, sleep disorders, and cognitive changes can occur for years before the disease progresses to the brain[148] and that Parkinson's disease is actually a multisystem disorder, not just a neurological ailment, which develops over a long period of time. According to the National Parkinson's Foundation, motor symptoms of Parkinson's disease only begin to manifest when most of the brain's dopamine-producing cells are already damaged.

Patients whose Parkinson's is diagnosed at an early stage have a better chance of slowing its progression. The most common approach to treating the disease is with oral intake of L-dopa, the chemical precursor to dopamine. But in some patients, long-term use of L-dopa will exacerbate PD symptoms. Unfortunately, there is no cure—yet.

Acclaimed neurologist Sir William Gowers was the first to mention cannabis as a treatment for tremors in 1888. In his *Manual of Diseases of the Nervous System,* Gowers noted that oral consumption of an "Indian hemp" extract quieted tremors temporarily, and after a year of chronic use, the patient's tremors nearly ceased.[149]

Modern scientific research supports the notion that cannabis could be beneficial in reducing inflammation and assuaging the symptoms of Parkinson's disease, as well as slowing its progression. Federally funded preclinical probes have documented the robust antioxidant and neuroprotective properties of CBD and THC with "particular application...in the treatment of neurodegenerative diseases, such as Alzheimer's disease, Parkinson's disease and HIV dementia." These findings formed the basis of a U.S. government patent, granted in 2003, on cannabinoids as antioxidants and neuroprotectants.[150]

More recently, scientists at the University of Louisville School of Medicine in Kentucky and the University of North Carolina at Greensboro have identified a previously unknown molecular target of CBD. In a presentation at the 2017 meeting of the International Cannabinoid Research Society in Montreal, they reported that CBD activates an orphan receptor in the brain called GPR6 in a way that boosts dopamine production.[151] This preclinical laboratory finding warrants further investigation given that as yet there is no cure for Parkinson's.

Though we don't know exactly what causes Parkinson's, one theory traces the earliest signs of Parkinson's to the enteric nervous system (the gut), the medulla (the brain stem), and the olfactory bulb in the brain, which controls one's sense of smell. New research shows that alterations in the microbiome may be a risk factor for Parkinson's[152] and related mitochondrial dysfunction[153] and energy depletion. This may be an underlying cause of the movement difficulties associated with Parkinson's disease.

Bacterial overgrowth in the small intestine has been linked to worsening motor function in patients with Parkinson's disease. In a 2017 article in the *European Journal of Pharmacology*, titled "The gut-brain axis in Parkinson's disease: Possibilities for food-based therapies,"[154] researchers examined the interplay between gut dysbiosis and Parkinson's. The authors report that "Parkinson's disease pathogenesis may be caused or exacerbated by dysbiotic microbiota-induced inflammatory responses...in the intestine and the brain."

As discussed previously, THC helps to maintain a well-balanced gut flora by contributing beneficial ("probiotic") bacteria, while CBD supports a healthy microbiome by enhancing endocannabinoid tone.

Post-Traumatic Stress Disorder

AS DESCRIBED IN Chapter 2, the cannabinoid receptor known as CB_1 mediates a broad range of physiological functions, including emotional learning, adapting to stress, and the ability to deactivate traumatic memories so that they feel less fresh and raw.

Chronic stress, however, boosts levels of the enzyme FAAH, which breaks down anandamide. When you have more FAAH, you have lower endocannabinoid levels. Endocannabinoid deficiency means poor CB_1 signaling. This results in a constant replaying of horrific situations, a hallmark of post-traumatic stress disorder (PTSD).

In 2012 a team of Brazilian scientists determined that chronic stress can decrease CB_1 receptor binding and expression particularly in the hippocampus, an area of the brain that plays a major role in short- and long-term memory consolidation.[155]

This process was brought into stark relief in a study published in *Psychoneuroendocrinology*, where a team of U.S. and Canadian scientists analyzed 46 men and women who were near the World Trade Center in New York City during the September 11 terrorist attacks. Twenty-four of these study participants suffered from PTSD following the attacks; 22 did not.[156]

The researchers found that people with PTSD had lower serum levels of the natural cannabinoid anandamide compared to those who did not show signs of PTSD after 9/11. In short, their endocannabinoid levels were low, skewing their CB_1 signaling and hindering their ability to "forget." The result: Those terrible memories were cemented in their brain.

"I Tried It"

Janelle Lassalle, 29,
Venice, California

As a person with PTSD and severe anxiety, Janelle Lassalle tried everything she could to better her health for many years with little success. "I tried everything: SSRIs, mood stabilizers, beta blockers, the whole nine yards," she said. "All of it somehow managed to make me even more ill." After feeling like pharmaceuticals had sucked the life from her, she tried CBD.

"CBD gave me my life back," Lassalle said. "It helped me stabilize my mood and manage neuropathic pain doctors hadn't been able to treat. Smoking CBD is also a much more natural and gentle alternative to using benzodiazepines for panic attacks, as they can be extremely habit forming."

After she started using CBD regularly, Lassalle noticed that she barely needed to take any medication to manage her symptoms of PTSD and anxiety. The oil has been a miracle for her health, given the previous amount of medication she used to require daily. "My use of benzos for panic attacks slipped down to virtually nothing," she said. "I didn't need pills for nightmares or insomnia anymore, either. I switched from using ibuprofen for pain too. I no longer need any mood-stabilizing medication of any kind."

Lassalle makes her own CBD oil–based tincture at home. Using CBD flower and organic avocado oil for her tincture blend, Lassalle takes the mixture up to three times per day. "This means holding it under my tongue for two minutes each time to allow full absorption," Lassalle said. "Sixty mg of CBD tends to be my usual dose, though I modify it as needed. Extreme anxiety requires higher doses. Travel anxiety for me is the worst, and when I travel, I typically take 100+ mg CBD. It's a dream."

CBD can help ease PTSD the same way it eases other anxiety disorders: CBD inhibits the absorption of anandamide and delays its metabolism by FAAH, so you have more of the mood-improving cannabinoid available to signal through the CB_1 receptor. Animal studies have also found that CBD reduces anxiety by binding directly to the 5HT1A serotonin receptor, which has an anxiolytic (antianxiety) effect.

In 2018, Brazilian researchers concluded, "Human and animal studies suggest that CBD may offer therapeutic benefits for disorders related to inappropriate responses to traumatic memories."[157] That's good news for those suffering from PTSD who have been through the worst stress life has to offer—combat, war, and other forms of extreme tragedy and violence.

It should also come as no surprise that since the late 1960s, many military veterans have turned to marijuana to self-medicate. In fact, lawmakers are finally pushing to help veterans have easier access to cannabis through H.R. 1647,[158] the Veterans Equal Access Act of 2019 (which was still in committee review process at the time of this writing),[159] allowing physicians to complete state legal medical marijuana–recommendation paperwork. Because of federal cannabis laws, Veterans Administration physicians are currently prohibited from doing this, and vets must turn to private out-of-network physicians.

> For those who can't legally access cannabis, hemp-derived CBD oil may be a viable option.

For those who can't legally access cannabis, hemp-derived CBD oil may be a viable option. People who reported taking CBD for PTSD in Project CBD's 2019 Survey said it was highly effective in addressing a range of symptoms, particularly anxiety, anger, irritability, depression, mood swings, and panic attacks. CBD also appeared to be helpful, though less so, in mitigating unwanted thoughts, nightmares, and heart palpitations in people with PTSD.

Psychosis and Schizophrenia

SCHIZOPHRENIA IS A mental disorder that affects a person's ability to think, feel, and behave clearly. It can cause psychotic episodes, and treatment is usually lifelong and involves antipsychotic medications with toxic side effects.

In 2012, researchers published a study in *Translational Psychiatry* showing that a CBD isolate can treat schizophrenia as effectively as antipsychotic pharmaceuticals—and with far fewer side effects.[160]

In this study, researchers led by Markus Leweke, MD, of the University of Cologne in Germany recruited 39 people with schizophrenia who were hospitalized for a psychotic episode. Nineteen of the study participants received an antipsychotic medication called amisulpride, while the other 20 were given CBD. After four weeks, both groups significantly improved. There was no difference in psychiatric symptoms between those getting CBD or amisulpride. But those taking CBD had fewer undesirable side effects, such as weight gain and movement disorders, compared to those taking amisulpride. The authors concluded, "These results suggest that cannabidiol is as effective at improving psychotic symptoms as the standard antipsychotic amisulpride."

CBD appears to provide antipsychotic relief by raising anandamide levels. Curiously, in an earlier study, Daniele Piomelli, PhD, director of the Center for the Study of Cannabis at the University of California in Irvine, discovered that people with schizophrenia had anandamide levels that were on average twice as high as mentally healthy people without the disorder.[161] Some scientists speculated that perhaps people with schizophrenia were essentially too high on elevated levels of their own endocannabinoids! But in reality, it seems that the brain actually increases anandamide levels to buffer stress and ease the symptoms of psychosis. The preponderance of evidence suggests that the higher the anandamide levels are in people with schizophrenia, the less severe their symptoms.

More recently, in 2020, researchers from Kings College in London used fMRI scans to monitor the brain activity of 13 people with psychosis while they performed a memory test after taking CBD or a placebo and compared it to 16 people without psychosis performing the same test. Those taking placebo had different brain activity in the prefrontal and mediotemporal brain areas associated with memory than the people without psychosis. When participants who had psychosis took one dose of CBD, their brain activity becomes more like their counterparts without the disease.

"Our study provides important insight into which areas of the brain CBD targets. It is the first time research has scanned the brains of people with a diagnosis of psychosis who have taken CBD and, although the sample is small, the results are compelling in that they demonstrate that CBD influences those very areas of the brain that have been shown to have unusual activity in people with psychosis," said the senior author on the study, Sagnik Bhattacharyya, MD, PhD.[162]

Importantly, in terms of cannabis and safety, one of the biggest health concerns and stigmas about cannabis use has been the idea that it can cause psychosis in vulnerable individuals. This has never been proven. It's worth noting that a 2012 meta-analysis published in *Schizophrenia Bulletin* showed that people diagnosed with schizophrenia who use cannabis function better cognitively than people with schizophrenia who do not use cannabis.[163]

Sleep Disorders

S LEEP DISORDERS ARE conditions that disturb your normal sleep patterns. Of the more than 80 recognized sleep disorders, difficulty falling or staying asleep is the most common. More than 50 million people in the United States suffer from chronic long-term sleep disorders each year, and an additional 20 to 30 million people experience occasional sleep problems.[164]

Prescription sleep medicines are known to have problematic side effects, so it's little wonder that people are increasingly turning to CBD and other alternatives to help them get a good night's rest. A national *Consumer Reports* survey reported that 10 percent of Americans who said they have tried CBD did so to help them sleep. And most who had tried it for better sleep said it helped.[165]

Similarly, Project CBD's 2019 survey showed favorable results with regard to sleep. Participants taking CBD for sleep were more likely to report having problems staying asleep than getting to sleep, though most people reported having difficulty with both. Participants said that CBD helped them get to sleep more quickly, reducing the average time it took to fall asleep from about an hour to 20 minutes. They also reported waking up much less often—1.4 times per night versus 4.3, or about a third as many times. Without CBD, almost three quarters of participants reported waking up tired; with CBD, only 9 percent did.[166]

In the case of serious sleep disorders like insomnia, relatively large doses appear to provide relief. In one study, people with insomnia who took 160 mg of pure CBD a day had an increase in their total sleep time and fewer nighttime awakenings.[167]

That said, CBD shouldn't be thought of as a "sleeping pill." It's not a barbiturate, nor is it soporific in the moderate doses that most people take. Instead it amplifies the natural signaling of the GABA-A receptor, which confers a relaxing effect. In other words, if you can't fall or stay asleep because your racing, anxious thoughts won't settle down enough to slumber, CBD may be your key to a restful night because it calms your mind.

Current research supports that theory. In a 2019 study published in the *Permanente Journal*, Colorado researchers investigated the health records of 72 men and women under psychiatric care who were given CBD (mostly 25 mg/day in capsule form, though a few people received higher doses) for anxiety and/or poor sleep.[168] After a month of CBD treatment, 79 percent reported improvements in anxiety and nearly 67 percent said they were enjoying better sleep. Results varied, however, as 15 percent and 25 percent experienced worsening symptoms in anxiety and sleep, respectively, possibly because of dosing issues. Also, while their anxiety levels remained lower over the three-month study period, their sleep scores fluctuated, and the benefits became milder.

"I Tried It"

Laura Dobratz, 31,
Minneapolis, Minnesota

L AYING AWAKE, staring at the ceiling, and counting sheep doesn't even begin to describe the agony of chronic insomnia. "I would have trouble sleeping pretty much every single night for years," Laura Dobratz, 31, says. "This meant I was always exhausted during the day and never felt well-rested, which took a toll on every aspect of my life."

Dobratz's insomnia began when her anxiety spiked during an extra stressful holiday season. It quickly turned into a vicious cycle of worrying, which made her unable to relax enough to fall asleep. The next day, this was followed by more anxiety because she wasn't sleeping.

Eventually, Dobratz sought out a psychiatrist to help with her anxiety. The doctor felt that they needed to treat her insomnia to see real improvement. The sleeping pills he prescribed helped her stay asleep, but she still had a tough time turning off the anxious part of her brain and falling asleep. So, her psychiatrist recommended she try CBD.

Dobratz opted for a broad-spectrum oil. "It costs a hundred dollars a bottle, but it's worth it because it works so well for me," she says. "It helps me chill out and not continuously worry about things when I'm trying to go to sleep. I'm so glad my psychiatrist recommended it, or I probably wouldn't have tried it." Plus, it doesn't have any lingering effects in the morning, unlike some sleeping medications, she adds.[169]

CBD may also help you get a better night's rest if you can't sleep because of chronic pain. A 2007 study found that up to 50 percent of 1,000 people with pain related to conditions like multiple sclerosis and cancer reported being able to attain good or very good sleep when taking Sativex (an oral spray medicine that is equal parts CBD and THC).[170] Similarly, a 2017 review of cannabinoid literature published in *Current Psychiatry Reports* reported that CBD-rich cannabis could improve sleep in people with chronic pain.[171]

Improved sleep is one of the most commonly mentioned benefits by people using CBD, and the benefits likely come from relieving other sleep-wrecking conditions like anxiety or pain. If you want to try CBD for sleep, it's worth noting that dosage may make a difference. Relatively larger doses appear to be sedative while smaller doses can have the opposite effect. A systematic review of the literature on CBD and humans published in 2012 in the journal *Pharmaceuticals* concluded that a daily CBD dose of 160 mg taken orally is potentially effective for sleep disorders, like insomnia, and that doses between 150 mg to 600 mg a day may have a sedative effect.[172] However, smaller doses of CBD may increase alertness and wakefulness.[173]

Traumatic Brain Injury and Stroke

T RAUMATIC BRAIN INJURY (TBI) is one of the leading causes of death worldwide in people under the age of 45.[174] Many who survive severe head injuries suffer permanent behavioral and neurological impairment that adversely impacts learning and memory and often requires long-term rehabilitation. An estimated 5.3 million Americans are living with a TBI-related disability.[175] Even so-called

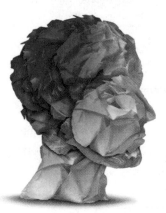

mild cases of TBI can result in post-traumatic seizures, impaired brain function, and lower life expectancy. People can also suffer an acquired or nontraumatic injury, such as in the case of stroke, which causes similar damage to the brain by internal factors like lack of blood flow and oxygen (ischemia).

Cannabinoids like THC and CBD may reduce the trauma and the symptoms that follow brain injury thanks to their positive interaction with the endocannabinoid system. A 2011 article in the *British Journal of Pharmacology* describes the ECS as "a self-protective mechanism" that kicks into high gear in response to a stroke or TBI. Coauthored by Israeli scientist Raphael Mechoulam, PhD, the article notes that endocannabinoid levels in the brain increase significantly during and immediately after a TBI. These endogenous compounds activate CB_1 and CB_2 receptors, which protect against TBI-induced neurological and motor deficits.[176]

By manipulating the endocannabinoid system with cannabinoids, medical scientists have been able to reduce brain injury in animal experiments. According to a 2010 report in the *British Journal of Pharmacology*, CBD can limit the amount of damaged tissue and help normalize the heart rhythm disturbances like arrhythmia that are common after a closed head injury.[177, 178]

CBD has been shown to reduce brain damage and improve functional recovery in animal studies of stroke and TBI.[179] A damaged brain can be remarkably plastic, but there is only a limited window of opportunity—generally thought of as 10 to 60 minutes[180]—for therapeutic intervention to prevent, attenuate, or delay the degenerative domino effect of brain cell death and damage to the protective blood-brain barrier that occurs during a secondary injury cascade (a wave of further damage that occurs as a result of the lack of blood flow to the brain following the initial injury).[181] CBD expands that window of opportunity. Researchers have learned that CBD can convey potent, long-lasting neuroprotection if given shortly before or as much as 12 hours after the onset of ischemia.[182] CBD has been shown to reduce brain damage and improve functional recovery in animal studies of stroke and TBI.[183]

In 2016, scientists at the University of Nottingham (UK) reported that CBD shields the protective blood-brain barrier from the damaging effects of lack of oxygen and fuel after an injury.[184] CBD prevents your blood-brain barrier from being damaged and becoming more permeable by activating the 5-HT1A serotonin receptor and the PPAR-gamma nuclear receptor.[185] CBD also protects the brain by increasing the concentration of endocannabinoids in the brain.

The researchers at the University of Nottingham have also conducted preclinical animal or laboratory research that examined the anti-inflammatory and neuroprotective effects of cannabidiolic acid (CBDA), the raw, unheated version of CBD found in the cannabis plant. "Like CBD," the researchers concluded, "CBDA is effective in reducing blood brain permeability and inflammation in a cellular model of stroke." CBD and CBDA both restore blood-brain barrier integrity by activating the 5-HT1A serotonin receptor, which mediates CBD's and CBDA's anti-inflammatory effects.[186]

Several athletes claim that CBD can help to ameliorate the lingering neurological problems associated with chronic traumatic encephalopathy (CTE), a particularly severe form of TBI caused by the accumulation of numerous concussions.[187] CTE increases the risk of neurological problems later in life and hastens the progression of dementia. The anecdotal benefits of CBD-rich cannabis oil for CTE are well known among football players, boxers, and other professional athletes who are prone to head injuries.

The 2019 Project CBD survey found that among people using CBD for a brain injury, CBD proved most helpful for relieving headaches, irritability, and agitation. CBD was less helpful for balance issues. In a small percentage of participants, CBD seemed to make issues with memory, concentration, and self-expression worse, but it's unclear if that was the result of CBD or THC or if there were other unknown factors at work.

Weight Issues: Obesity, Anorexia, and Cachexia

IT'S NO SECRET that weight is a national fixation. Most of the scale obsession focuses on weight loss, as obesity levels continue to rise around the world. There's evidence that CBD may help with obesity and related issues. Cannabis may also be helpful for cachexia (loss of weight and appetite in someone who is not actively trying to lose weight) and anorexia (an emotional disorder characterized by obsession with weight loss and refusal to eat).

With regard to overweight and obesity, there are many theories as to why the population has grown heavier and people struggle to lose weight and keep it off. Certainly diet and lack of exercise play a role, but so does our endocannabinoid system (which, of course, is also connected to and influenced by our diet and exercise habits). And there's growing evidence that CBD may be able to improve metabolism and assist with weight loss by rebalancing the ECS and priming the gut-brain axis.

CBD may help you eat less by reducing your appetite.

In fact, classic weight-loss strategies like diet and exercise may work in part by improving cannabinoid receptor signaling, according to Brazilian scientists at the Federal University of São Paulo.[188] As we learned in Chapter 4, exercise improves endocannabinoid tone. So does a healthy diet low in sugar and carbs and rich in leafy greens, polyphenols, probiotics, essential fatty acids, and high-fiber foods. And that, in turn, helps with weight loss.

There's also evidence that CBD may help you eat less by reducing your appetite.[189] Whereas THC is well known to cause hunger (aka the munchies), by stimulating CB_1 receptors, CBD does not. In fact, CBD may trigger a molecular response that reduces appetite.[190] A 2012 study found that rats given CBD ate significantly less when offered food. But such studies have not yet been done on humans.[191]

Interestingly, though THC does appear to stimulate appetite, marijuana users as a demographic are less obese and are less likely to develop metabolic syndrome than nonusers, according to a study of nearly 8,500 adults ages 20 to 59 conducted by scientists at the University of Miami in Florida, published in the *American Journal of Medicine*.[192] Several factors may contribute to this curious but noteworthy finding. While cannabis is notorious for causing "the munchies" by stimulating the CB_1 receptor, THC also activates CB_2 receptors in a way that balances and improves overall endocannabinoid tone. And THC, a probiotic compound, may also promote metabolic health by fostering beneficial gut bacteria.

It appears that CBD also stimulates fat burning. There are different types of fat that behave very differently in your body. There's the white stuff, which we know as the bumps and bulges that sit underneath our skin and not only acts as stored energy but also produces hormones that can disrupt healthy feelings of hunger and satiety. Then there's brown fat; this is the type of fat you actually want more of because it's metabolically active and helps burn white fat. There's even beige fat, which is white fat that acts like brown fat. Overweight people have proportionately less brown and beige fat than their leaner counterparts.

Research published in *Molecular and Cellular Biochemistry* concluded that CBD plays a role in "fat browning," meaning it helps the body convert white fat into weight-reducing brown fat and assists in breaking down fats more efficiently. CBD also lowers insulin resistance and promotes normal sugar metabolism. All of these benefits can make it easier to attain and maintain healthy weight. So while there is still a lot to learn, CBD is promising for weight loss and 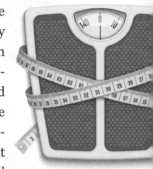 in the treatment of obesity.[193, 194] But it's important to remember that CBD is a supplement to healthy active living. You will likely see more benefits from adding it to your general health and/or weight-loss plan if you are also eating well and exercising.

On the other side of the spectrum from unwanted weight gain is cachexia—unwanted weight loss and muscle wasting, which is a common side effect of diseases like cancer, AIDS, obstructive pulmonary disease, and hormonal deficiency. Cachexia is among the conditions that Pal Pacher, MD, PhD, and George Kunas, MD, PhD, leading scientists with the U.S. National Institutes of Health, listed that could be helped by modulating the endocannabinoid system.[195] Since the ECS helps regulate appetite, and activating CB_1 receptors can stimulate appetite, cannabis products offer some hope for treating cachexia and anorexia.[196]

Unchecked, cachexia can lead to anemia and weakness to the point of immobility. The wasting syndrome was one of the telltale signs of HIV infection, and it was also one of the main reasons why many people with AIDS embraced cannabis as a therapeutic when the AIDS epidemic exploded in the 1980s. More than any other single factor, it was the AIDS crisis that made access to cannabis an urgent, cutting-edge issue in California, leading to the legalization of medical marijuana in 1996. Today cannabis is allowed for the treatment of cachexia in many U.S. states where medical marijuana is legal.

Anorexia has one of the highest death rates of any psychiatric condition. THC is a well-known appetite stimulant, and studies on THC and dronabinol (a synthetic form of pure THC) showed that both helped people with anorexia gain some weight.[197] Though most of the scientific attention has centered on THC for its appetite-stimulating abilities, cannabis, especially CBD-rich cannabis, may have greater therapeutic value than THC alone, which has been available by prescription since 1985. Adding CBD to the mix may provide additional benefits since anorexia is a complex condition that also involves anxiety and obsession, both of which may benefit from CBD.

Women's Health

Since CBD can help with pain, sleep, and mood disturbances, it makes sense that women would be drawn to CBD products for relief from menstrual cramps, PMS, and symptoms associated with menopause, such as mood swings, sleep disturbances, temperature regulation, and altered brain function.

The endocannabinoid system can be dysregulated during menopause, so it's logical to consider that fortifying and balancing the ECS with cannabinoids like CBD could relieve uncomfortable symptoms. Currently, there's very little research in this area. The same holds true for symptoms surrounding the menstrual cycle

"I Tried It"

Aliza Sherman Risdahl,
55, Anchorage, Alaska

FOR YEARS, ALIZA SHERMAN Risdahl, 55, has been going through menopause. She has also been struggling with anxiety and arthritis in her neck.

"I initially tried cannabis with THC to help alleviate both anxiety and pain (I live in a state where cannabis is legal), and while it was extremely effective and helpful, I worried about being altered in any way that I couldn't be at my most productive," Risdahl said. "My work as a writer and marketing consultant revolves around my brain being sharp, so when I learned that full-spectrum CBD could be helpful for anxiety and pain, I tried it and found it to be effective."

When she started taking CBD, Risdahl noticed a complete change in her moods. "It relieves anxiety and reduces irritability," Risdahl said. "It also seems to regulate my hormones so my [menopause] symptoms have been less severe."

In addition to taking CBD oil, Risdahl also uses CBD topicals. These two in combination have really helped relieve the arthritis in her neck—so much that she's nearly eliminated use of over-the-counter pain medications. "I haven't had to take any ibuprofen since taking CBD and have not had to resort to any pain medications," Risdahl said. "For anxiety, it is hard to fully gauge the effectiveness as I'm dealing with many stressors in my life, but I do feel that if I were not taking CBD, my reactions to the stress would be more severe."

Risdahl makes sure to tell her doctors that she is on CBD, and so far, none have shown any concern. Like most doctors, they are glad that the oil has impacted her life in such positive ways. "I always tell every doctor that I use CBD," Risdahl said. "So far, none of them have known very much about CBD, but because I am not currently on any other medications, it has not been an issue."

like PMS. However, there is certainly some research showing CBD alleviates individual symptoms, especially sleep disturbances and mood, and there is a growing body of anecdotal evidence.

In Project CBD's 2019 survey, among people taking CBD for PMS, menopause, or other female hormonal conditions, CBD appeared to be highly effective in addressing mood disturbances and pain. It also appears to help mitigate night sweats and, to a lesser degree, hot flashes associated with menopause. CBD was less effective at ameliorating the bloating common to menstruation; and users found that it wasn't as helpful for alleviating sexual discomfort, low sex drive, and dry skin associated with menopause.[198]

CBD may also help manage endometriosis, a condition in which the endometrium (the tissue that normally lines the uterus) grows outside of the uterus. This can cause debilitating pain during periods, pain during intercourse, and can lead to infertility. Women with endometriosis have lower levels of CB_1 receptors in their endometrium. According to a 2017 study, this suggests that reduced endocannabinoid system function may lead to the growth of the tissue outside the uterus as well as to a more severe pain experience.[199]

> CBD may also help manage endometriosis.

That means balancing the endocannabinoid system with cannabinoids may not only help relieve the pain associated with endometriosis but also help mitigate the underlying causes of the condition, say the researchers who concluded, "Targeting endocannabinoid modulation to treat pain is probably more than just treating the pain as it may impact several levels of the pathogenesis and the proliferation of the disease."

Finally, as mentioned on page 77, CBD may be a particularly potent ally against certain types of breast cancer cells. Most recently, in a 2019 study published in the *International Journal of Molecular Sciences*, a team of Slovakian and Austrian researchers concluded that cannabinoids like CBD and THC "may decelerate tumor progression in breast cancer patients" and that cannabinoids "are not only active against estrogen receptor positive, but also estrogen-resistant breast cancer cells."[200]

For information on CBD and pregnancy, see page 188.

3

The CBD User's Guide

S O NOW YOU have a better idea about what CBD is, how it works with your endocannabinoid system, and the dozens of diseases and conditions it could help, as well as how it can keep you happier and healthier. The big question that likely remains in your mind is "How should I use it?"

We are here to bring you that information because we know figuring out how to use CBD, how much to take, and how to choose a product can be complicated. Unlike vitamins that have Daily Recommended Allowances or over-the-counter pills with clear directions, CBD can feel like a bit of a mystery.

There are myriad reasons for that:
- Federal law limits what manufacturers and doctors can say;
- Different types of CBD produce different effects;
- Many factors, including your weight, gender, age, and genetics, influence how you'll respond to CBD; and
- CBD works on a bell curve, so small and large doses may actually have opposite effects.

That's a lot of information to process, which is what this section is all about, starting with the basics of how CBD is made, what forms you can buy it in, and how to choose the type and delivery method that is right for you and your personal CBD needs.

You'll find an entire chapter on buying CBD. Because CBD is unregulated, there is an awful lot of snake oil sitting on the market alongside scientifically sound products. You'll learn what goes into a quality CBD product, where the best CBD comes from, and how to know a good product when you see one.

We cut through the confusion on CBD product ingredients and concentrations. You'll learn why "pure" CBD isn't usually the best CBD and how to confidently read a label so you're buying what you want.

There is also an entire chapter devoted to dosing, which may require a little trial and error to get exactly right. You'll find the facts on each form of CBD: how quickly it works, how long it lasts, what it's best for, and what a typical dose looks like. We provide a personal action planner so you can pick, plot, and track your CBD usage to dial in your optimum personal dose.

CBD is very safe, but there are some precautions to know about, especially with regard to special populations like children and pregnant women. We have those covered, as well as how to avoid problematic interactions with common over-the-counter and prescription drugs.

Plus, there's a complete recipe section for those who would like to make their own CBD balms, skin creams, and even tinctures, including special recipes to help with sleep, stress, inflammation, and pain.

Finally, because pets are part of the family—and all mammals have an endocannabinoid system that keeps them healthy—there's a special section devoted to CBD for your furry companions. You'll learn the difference between CBD for people and CBD for pets, what to look for in CBD pet products, and, of course, how to find the right dose for your pet's needs.

6

How CBD Oil is Made

I F YOU WANT to buy quality CBD, it's helpful to know something about where it came from and how it was extracted from the plant and made into a product. Where CBD-rich hemp plants are grown can influence the quality of the product. Boutique cannabis growers talk about *terroir* in much the same way as vintners talk about the unique qualities of soil where grapes are grown. Soil quality is especially important since hemp is known to be a sponge for chemicals in the soil.

Different manufacturers use different methods to extract CBD from the cannabis plant, and the way it is extracted, processed, and refined has a large impact on the quality and purity of the product. With advances in nanotechnology, cannabis oil manufacturers can even create water-soluble versions of CBD for inclusion in beverages and "mocktails" (nonalcoholic medical cocktails).

As described in Part I, CBD is one of more than 100 unique cannabinoids found in the oily resin of the cannabis plant. That sticky, gooey resin is concentrated on the dense clusters of cannabis flowers, commonly called *buds*, which are covered by tiny, mushroom-shaped cannabinoid factories called *trichomes*. There are two broad categories of cannabis plants: industrial hemp plants with skimpy, low-resin flowers; and medicinal or drug plants with many resinous flowers.

Trichomes are sort of like the plant's lymph glands—they produce and pump out medicinal compounds, including CBD, THC, and various aromatic terpenes to protect the plant from getting injured or sick. The oily resin guards the plant from heat and ultraviolet radiation. It has antifungal, antibacterial, and insecticidal properties that deter bugs, birds, and other animals from eating the plant. The stickiness of the resin provides another defensive layer by trapping bugs. The cannabinoids and terpenes in that resin also show

> Trichomes are sort of like the plant's lymph glands.

promise in treating and managing the symptoms of a broad range of human diseases.

As far as medicinal and recreational cannabis goes, the resin is where the action is. In addition to the resin-rich trichomes found mainly on the plant's odiferous flowers and to a lesser extent on the leaves, there are also tiny trichomes, which dot the stalk of the plant. These contain hardly any resin.

Companies that say they extract CBD from resin-deficient hemp stalk are most likely making false claims (though some may say this simply to avoid oversight by the FDA or other government regulators).

Sources of CBD Oil

To make CBD products, manufacturers extract the oil from the resinous trichomes of cannabis plants. There are many different cannabis strains or varietals. The amount of CBD present in the trichomes will depend on the particular variety of cannabis or hemp that's been grown specifically for CBD oil extraction. The more resinous trichomes in the flower tops, the more CBD there is to extract.

The best source of CBD oil is organically grown, high-resin, CBD-rich cannabis that tips the scales at 20 percent CBD by dry weight. But these varieties typically have a little more THC than the legal limit for hemp as ordained by the Farm Bill. The challenge for hemp farmers is to grow high-resin plants with as much CBD as possible without exceeding 0.3 percent THC.

Low-resin industrial hemp grown for fiber or seed oil (as distinct from the essential oil, which is a concentrated mixture extracted from the flowers and leaves) is not an optimal source of CBD for several reasons:

- Industrial hemp typically contains far less cannabidiol (between 1 percent and 3.5 percent CBD by dry weight) compared to high-resin, CBD-rich cannabis.[1] So, a large amount of industrial hemp is required to extract a relatively small amount of CBD. This raises the risk of contaminants. Hemp is a bioaccumulator; the plant naturally draws toxins from the soil. That's a great benefit for farmers wanting to clean polluted soil, but it's not so great for making ingestible medicinal oil products. Oil extracted from hemp and cannabis will concentrate the toxins as well as the healing compounds.[2]

- Until recently, CBD oil was often a byproduct or afterthought product of industrial hemp grown primarily for other purposes, like textiles and seed oil (which is not the same as CBD oil). Farmers can make additional money if they sell their unused hemp biomass to a business that wants to extract CBD from the leftover plant matter. This dual-use practice is widespread and barely regulated, if at all, and the hemp biomass is often tainted with residues of pesticides and toxic solvents used to extract the CBD oil.

- Low-resin industrial hemp lacks the robust mix of medicinal terpenes and secondary cannabinoids found in high-resin cannabis.[3] The therapeutic benefits of CBD and THC are enhanced by the entourage effect, as we described in Chapter 1.

It won't always be possible to find out which varieties of cannabis plants were the source of the CBD in the products you buy, but some products will list or advertise this information. Unfortunately, false claims are common in the unregulated CBD marketplace; but, in general, look for products made by companies that freely provide as much information as possible. See Chapter 8 for more tips on how to find quality CBD products.

How CBD Is Extracted from Cannabis

The purpose of an extraction is to make CBD and other beneficial components of the plant available in a highly concentrated form. After it is extracted from the plant and the solvent is removed, the CBD oil may be refined and formulated into a variety of products—edibles, tinctures, gel caps, vape oil cartridges, topicals, beverages, and more.

Extracting CBD-rich oil and processing can be a painstaking process. When you separate CBD from the plant material, it produces a viscous, potent oil. The texture and purity of the oil depend largely on the method used to extract and refine it. There are several ways to extract CBD oil from cannabis, with each method having its pros and cons. Some are safer and more effective than others.

CO_2 Extraction

Carbon dioxide (CO_2) extraction is one of the most commonly used commercial methods to extract CBD from the plant. It's also one of the safest methods not just for the people doing the extraction but also for the end consumer, because it doesn't rely on toxic solvents to extract CBD oil. That means there will less likely be impurities in the final product. At room temperature, carbon dioxide is a gas; but at high pressure and fluctuating temperature, CO_2 becomes a liquid while maintaining the fluid dynamics of a gas. This is known as a supercritical state. In that state, the CO_2 acts as a solvent and flushes out the active ingredients from the plant.

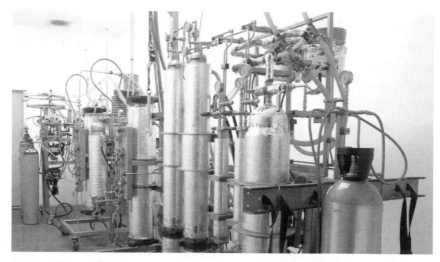

The supercritical CO2 extraction method uses carbon dioxide under high pressure and shifting temperatures to isolate, preserve, and maintain the purity of medicinal CBD oil.

Using this method, a skillful operator can fine-tune the extraction process by changing the temperature and/or pressure slightly in this *supercritical state*. As the pressure drops, a crude, waxy, CBD-rich substance, golden in color, separates from the gas and deposits into a collection vessel. Afterward, the golden oil undergoes a process known as winterization, which filters out the plant waxes to leave a safe, clean, CBD-rich oil.

Supercritical CO_2 extraction is not simple or cheap. Manufacturers need to invest in expensive equipment that requires a well-trained technician to operate, but it yields a high-quality CBD-rich product—all the more so when the oil is extracted from high-resin, trichome-dense cannabis flower.

Ethanol Extraction

CBD is soluble in alcohol, and there's a long history of using food-grade ethanol (aka grain alcohol) to extract medicinal compounds from cannabis and other plants. Dating back to 1850, the U.S. Pharmacopeia

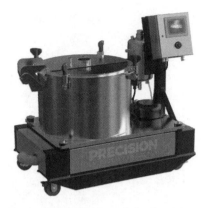

The C-40 Centrifuge made by Precision Extraction Solutions is used to extract CBD with ethanol.

(an official, nongovernment-affiliated publication of medicinal drugs with their effects and directions for use) recommended ethanol-based tinctures of "Indian hemp" (otherwise known as "gunjah," or *Cannabis indica*, a drug plant) to treat numerous ailments, including neuralgia, depression, hemorrhage, pain, and muscle spasm.[4]

These tinctures were a standard part of American health care until shortly after the passage of the Marihuana Tax Act in 1937, a law grounded more in public resentment of Mexican immigrants than in public health. By requiring a prohibitive tax on all marijuana transactions, Congress in effect made all forms of cannabis consumption de facto illegal. Of course, some people in marginalized Mexican American communities still made their own home-brewed cannabis tinctures, but that was strictly an underground practice.

Now, with the growing interest in CBD oil, ethanol extraction of cannabis oil is back above ground and becoming more popular. Today, many manufacturers are using food-grade grain alcohol as a solvent to create very potent, high-quality CBD-rich oil extracts. The one downside is that ethanol also efficiently pulls chlorophyll out from the plant, so the end product might be grassy or bitter tasting.

Often sold in plastic, needleless syringes to make dosing and administration a little easier, ethanol extracts should contain a concentrated version of the essential oil derived from whole-plant cannabis, including all the cannabinoids and the other medicinal components. This means that a small amount of THC will also be present in a CBD-rich ethanol extraction.

As with supercritical oil extractions, this type of CBD product can be quite potent, so it's best to "start low and go slow," meaning start with a small dose and give it time to work before taking more. The same holds true for any cannabis oil concentrate.

Hydrocarbon Extraction

Another way to extract CBD oils is through a process called *hydrocarbon extraction*. Manufacturers using this method will typically use hydrocarbons like butane, hexane, or propane to strip out the cannabinoids and terpenes from raw cannabis. The hydrocarbons are then removed, leaving behind the extract.

When performed properly, this type of extraction can be a very effective way of separating cannabinoids and terpenes from the plant.

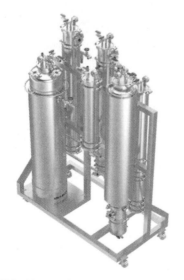

N.B. Oler Engineering manufactures several types of machines for CBD extraction, including this hydrocarbon extraction device.

Because hydrocarbon extraction doesn't involve heating the plant matter, it can preserve CBD in its raw, natural form, known as CBDA (cannabidiolic acid), which has unique medicinal properties of its own, especially with regard to treating nausea. When CBDA is heated, it loses its "A" and turns into CBD.

But hydrocarbon extraction has its drawbacks and can be dangerous. The problem is that butane and other hydrocarbons are highly flammable solvents, and residue from these toxic solvents can damage your brain cells.[5] If these solvents aren't fully purged from the CBD oil extract, their consumption can be harmful—especially for someone with a compromised immune system. Unfortunately, without access to reliable lab test results, there's no way to tell if these solvents have been fully purged. So, if you have a compromised immune system, your best bet is to look for products made with CBD extracted by a safer method.

Types of CBD-Rich Oil Extracts

After CBD oil is extracted, it's refined and processed into one of the thousands of CBD products on the market. There are many different ways to take CBD, which we'll explain in more detail in the next chapter. But generally, all CBD products will be classified as either CBD isolates, broad-spectrum CBD oil with no THC, or full-spectrum oil with a tiny amount of THC (no more than 0.3 percent). And if medical cannabis is legal in your state, you also might be able to access regulated CBD-rich cannabis products (with varying amounts of THC) that are sold in licensed dispensaries. (See "The State of Legal Cannabis," page 16). Here's what those product designations mean:

Do-It-Yourself CBD

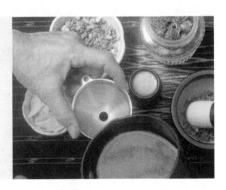

CBD dissolves in oil, so you can make your own CBD product at home. MCT (medium-chain triglyceride) oil is a widely used carrier oil for both topical and edible use, but other oils work, too. See page 216 for a topical oil recipe and page 222 for an edible oil recipe.

Full-spectrum CBD: The product will say full spectrum on the label. It is also sometimes called "whole plant," meaning that the product contains the concentrated version of the full essential oil with the

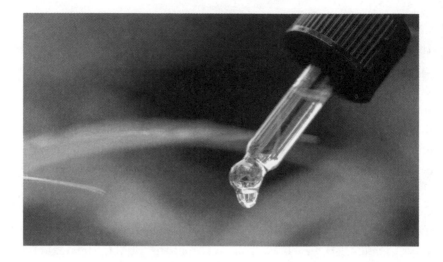

same CBD:THC ratio that's present in the whole-plant matrix. If it's a hemp-derived CBD product, the label should clearly indicate that the product contains <0.3 percent THC, as required by federal law.

Broad-spectrum CBD: Broad-spectrum CBD-rich oil is basically the essential oil from cannabis minus the THC. Broad-spectrum oil is created by removing the THC from essential oil extracted from cannabis. The product label should clearly indicate that it is 0 percent THC or THC-Free. Some manufacturers mix a CBD isolate with small amounts of other cannabinoids and terpenes (but no THC) in a carrier medium to create a faux broad-spectrum entourage. It's not as effective as a true broad-spectrum oil but still gives you more of an entourage effect than CBD isolates.

CBD isolate: An isolate means just CBD, nothing else from the plant. The product should be clearly labeled as isolate. Some products will also be labeled as 99 percent or 100 percent pure CBD. These products may contain other carrier ingredients like oils (often pressed hemp seed oil) to create tinctures without other cannabis molecules like THC, terpenes, and various other cannabinoids. Also, you can buy CBD isolate powder from various online storefronts. This is a fine crystalline powder from which all the other hemp plant matter, including oils, terpenes, chlorophyll, and more, have been stripped, leaving pure CBD behind. You can try mixing it into food or drink or putting some in a capsule.

CBD distillate: You may also come across something called a CBD distillate. Distillates are essentially a cocktail of different isolates and contain upward of 80 percent CBD along with small amounts of other cannabinoids and terpenes.

CBD-rich medical cannabis: This book is primarily dedicated to CBD products. This includes a major subset of cannabis products that many people find extremely beneficial but that are not legal in every state and remain illegal on the federal level. These are considered medical marijuana products (not hemp) because they exceed the 0.3 percent THC limit. Licensed dispensaries in states that have legalized marijuana for therapeutic and/or recreational use may sell a variety of CBD-rich products, including tinctures, topicals, edibles, flowers, and vaping liquids that are high in CBD and relatively low in THC. If you're 21 or older and you live in a state with legal access to cannabis, you can visit your local dispensary to find a broad range of CBD-rich products with varying ratios of CBD and THC.

Water-Soluble CBD Products

Cannabinoids like CBD are sticky, waxy chemicals. They like to mix with oil, not water. Because CBD is fat soluble, it is also less easily absorbed in the human body, which is about 65 percent water.

Some manufacturers are trying to address this issue by creating cannabinoid products that dissolve in water. One way to make cannabinoids water soluble is to create an emulsion (tiny particles of one liquid suspended in another) of the cannabinoid (either CBD or THC) and coat it in a surfactant to stabilize it. So, essentially, the individual molecules of CBD or THC are trapped in "molecular cages" that dissolve in water and are easily broken down and absorbed by the body.

Hemp Seed Oil

Sometimes misleadingly referred to as "hemp oil," hemp seed oil is not the same as CBD-rich oil extracted from the flowers and leaves of the plant. Oil pressed from hemp seed contains no CBD, no THC, no plant cannabinoids to speak of; but it's great for making varnish, paint, soap, nutraceuticals, and much more. Protein-rich hemp seed oil contains omega-3 fatty acids and other healthful compounds. You'll find protein powder derived from hemp seed at your local community market. It's a great dietary supplement.

Because these products are easier for your body to absorb, they will take effect more quickly (perhaps as quickly as 20 minutes) compared to a lipophilic oil-based CBD product. Because of its enhanced bioavailability, water-soluble CBD may pack a stronger punch than the same amount of regular CBD. But there's a trade-off, as water-soluble CBD will also have a shorter duration of effect.

The process of solubilizing CBD and/or THC can reverse over time, so brands that develop water-soluble formulations need to ensure the stability of their products so that the CBD doesn't stick to the side of the can.

7

What Is the Best Way to Take CBD?

YOU CAN CONSUME CBD in a wide array of products and forms, including capsules, tinctures, edibles, balms, and vaping devices. Everybody processes cannabinoids a little differently and has different reasons for using CBD, which means that finding your ideal form of consumption may take some experimentation.

When deciding where to start, consider the following factors:

Onset: How quickly will the cannabinoids in the product begin to work?

Dose: How much do you need to take?

Distribution: Which parts of your body will be most affected?

Duration: How long will the effects last?

Calculating dosage depends on the quality and potency of the product and the reason for using it. This will be discussed in Chapter 9.

Here's what you need to know about the various ways to take CBD.[5]

Under-the-Tongue/Sublingual and Oral-Mucosal Tinctures

Traditionally, when we think of "taking medicine," we think of swallowing a teaspoon or capful of liquid (often as quickly as we can because medicine often tastes bad). With CBD, one of the most common (and effective) ways is not swallowing per se, but holding the liquid in your mouth, particularly under your tongue, for a minute or so, so the active ingredients can be absorbed there before you swallow it and send it through your digestive system. This is known as *sublingual* or *oral-mucosal* administration. The liquid is usually a tincture, a medicine that can be made by steeping a plant in alcohol.

Onset: 15 minutes to an hour.

Dose: 2.5 to 5 mg CBD is a common starting dose if the tincture includes some THC. When using CBD-rich cannabis, this delivery method could cause a slight high in new users, depending on how much THC is in the product. A CBD-infused tincture without THC typically requires a higher starting dose (up to 25 mg).

Distribution: Absorbed through the mouth into the bloodstream, where it then distributes evenly throughout the body.

Duration: After 6 to 9 hours, most of the CBD and/or THC will have been metabolized or eliminated from the body.

Oral-mucosal tinctures are absorbed directly into the blood vessels in the mouth and under the tongue. Bypassing digestion also means less of it is broken down through the digestive process, so sublingual products have a considerably higher bioavailability than edible CBD products—with between 13 and 19 percent and maybe up to 35 percent, according to some research, entering your bloodstream.[6, 7] The relative quick action and long duration of oral-mucosal tinctures make them suitable for many chronic conditions.

These usually come in one of two forms: an under-the-tongue spray or a dropper with a marking at a specific volume (usually 0.5

mL or 1.0 mL). This allows for consistent, measurable dosing.

After spraying the liquid or dropping it under the tongue, you should try to wait at least 1 minute before swallowing. Some manufacturers suggest swishing CBD oil around in your mouth before swallowing to increase surface contact. Effects usually start after 15 to 30 minutes and peak around an hour and a half after taking it.

Tinctures typically involve a solvent like ethanol oil. Some of the adverse side effects, like diarrhea, attributed to cannabis extracts may actually be due to repeated ingestion of the carrier oil.

Although sublingual sprays can provide rapid and precise dosing, they can be confusing for patients. If you spray CBD oil under the tongue but then swallow immediately, your body will process it like an edible. This means that it will take longer to have an effect. And if there's THC in the tincture, people may take another dose after half an hour, thinking they hadn't had enough, which could lead to accidental intoxication.

Finally, be prepared: Some full-spectrum CBD-rich oil products, depending on how they are formulated, could have an earthy, somewhat bitter, almost grassy flavor. It goes away quickly, but initially it

Nasal Mists

One of the newer methods for consuming CBD is nasal mist spray. These products may come in regular or extra strength, delivering 1 mg or 2 mg of CBD per spray respectively. Nasal mists are similar to saline sinus solutions and medicines that you take through your sinus passages. CBD delivered via a nasal spray reaches the bloodstream quickly. In theory, you can use it discreetly almost anywhere without worrying about potential long-term lung health concerns posed by smoking and vaping. But this delivery method has yet to catch on among CBD consumers, and it's too early to say how well they work or how long they last.

can be quite strong. Some people don't mind it and even like it, while others find it a bit unpleasant.

Edibles and Capsules

Eating CBD in the form of gummies, chocolates, and/or pills is another popular way to take CBD. Because it needs to pass through the digestive system, oral ingestion is not generally the best mode for fast, acute relief or action. But it can deliver deeper, more sustained relief compared to other modes of administration.

Onset: 1 to 2 hours.

Dose: Doses of orally consumed CBD-rich products range from 5 mg to hundreds of milligrams. When using full-spectrum CBD-rich products with THC, the threshold for mild psychoactive effects is 3 mg THC in most new users.

Distribution: Absorbed through the gut and modified in the liver, after which it spreads fairly evenly throughout the body.

Duration: THC's psychoactive effects subside after about 6 hours in most people; other therapeutic effects may last up to 12 hours.

Ingested cannabinoids are absorbed through the intestines and sent to the liver. It takes about an hour to feel the effects when taken on an empty stomach or up to 2 hours (and sometimes longer) with food. If using a cannabis or hemp product with a combination of CBD and THC, avoid redosing edibles for at least 3 hours after taking the initial dose.

On the way to the liver, plant cannabinoids will interact with receptors in the gut, so the effect on conditions like irritable bowel syndrome and other inflammatory conditions will be more pronounced with oral ingestion. Once in the liver, several enzymes will start to modify CBD and THC in a process called *first-pass metabolism*.[8] Note that orally consumed THC is largely converted to 11-OH-THC, which is a metabolized version of THC that actually causes a stronger high than THC itself. This, along with the long

CBD-Infused Beverages

With advances in nano-technology, cannabis oil manufacturers have been able to create water-soluble versions of CBD for inclusion in beverages, such as iced teas, soft drinks, coffee, cocktails, and "mocktails" (nonalcoholic medical cocktails).

Nanotech facilitates liquid homogenization, a process for reducing a substance into extremely small particles that are more easily distributed throughout a fluid, and makes them more bioavailable (better absorbed in your body) than their oily, naturally occurring counterparts. But there are major trade-offs that may cancel some of the advantages of this type of nanoemulsified single-molecule CBD. Nanoemulsified CBD may be easier to absorb systemically, but it also metabolizes much quicker, thereby reducing the duration of its effect.

Two CBD-infused beverages to be leery of are coffee and cocktails, as the benefits of CBD may be overridden by the downsides of the other chemicals found in these drinks.

CBD-infused coffee is often marketed as a way to avoid the caffeine jitters, but how does CBD actually affect caffeine's stimulating properties?

Caffeine and CBD have opposing actions via the neurotransmitter adenosine. Adenosine, an endogenous anti-inflammatory compound, binds to specific A2A receptors to slow down your nerve cell activity and make you feel drowsy. Caffeine acts as an antagonist that blocks adenosine from binding to the A2A receptor; hence, the energy uplift from a cup of Joe.

When caffeine attaches to the adenosine receptor, instead of slowing down, the nerves speed up. CBD has the opposite effect—it inhibits and delays the re-uptake and breakdown of adenosine, leaving more in your system. In this push and pull involving adenosine, caffeine will likely overpower and override the relaxing effects of CBD.

Finally, CBD may be the most sought after ingredient for any cocktail mixologist worth their salt not only because it's the hot new ingredient on the block but also because research shows CBD may protect the liver, which alcohol is known to damage. Animal studies have found that CBD can protect against alcohol-induced fatty liver disease by promoting the turnover of new cells and tissue regeneration.[9] Those results have not been shown in humans, however, and it's not clear that adding CBD to an occasional cocktail will make much of a difference in terms of one's health, though it may instill a false sense of security and encourage people to drink more than they normally would. CBD-infused rum is still rum, and there's no good reason to combine CBD with distilled spirits.

Health tip: Making your own CBD tea can effectively deliver CBDA (CBD in its raw form, which has medicinal properties of its own). The water used to make tea generally isn't hot enough to break it down. Just add a small piece of raw hemp or cannabis flower to a favorite cup of steeping tea. You might not enjoy the taste of pure cannabis tea, as the flavor will likely be too harsh.

duration of edibles, is why new users should become comfortable with THC's psychoactive effects before using cannabis edibles that contain more than 5 mg THC.

Eating a well-made edible is an easy way to take CBD and can mask the earthy flavor some find unpleasant. The longer-lasting effect of edibles and capsules makes them suitable for many chronic conditions.

Inhaling CBD

Smoking and vaping are fast, efficient ways to get CBD into your system. The primary consideration when using this method to consume CBD is lung health, so it is imperative to choose products carefully.

Onset: Seconds to minutes.

Dose: As little as a single puff may be sufficient. A typical joint includes 0.3 to 1.0 g of cannabis. How much CBD you get in a preroll (a cannabis cigarette) depends upon the particular plant variety present in the preroll. A joint made with CBD-rich hemp or cannabis could contain around 50 to 150 mg CBD per joint.

Distribution: Affects the lungs immediately, then the heart and brain, after which it is distributed fairly evenly throughout the body.

Duration: Most effects, including psychoactivity, subside after 2 to 3 hours.[10]

Smoking CBD

Obviously, there's nothing new about smoking cannabis-based products, as people around the world have been smoking cannabis flower for a long time. In some states, you can buy hemp flower CBD buds and roll your own joints. Or you can buy what are called *prerolls,* which are just as they sound: CBD-rich cannabis rolled into a joint that contains less than 0.3 percent THC. Prerolls are ready for smoking, a convenience that appeals to many consumers.

Inhalation is the fastest method for administering cannabis-based

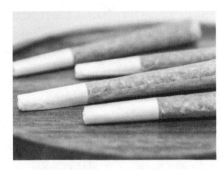

CBD prerolls

products. When CBD and other cannabinoids are heated and inhaled through the lungs, they cross the blood-brain barrier before getting metabolized by the liver. Usually, between 20 percent to 30 percent (and maybe more) of the phytocannabinoids like CBD and THC are absorbed this way. The heat from either smoking or vaporizing cannabis converts the acid cannabinoids (CBDA and THCA) into their neutral forms of CBD and THC.

The speedy onset and relatively short duration make inhalation an appropriate response to acute problems. People might choose to smoke or vape CBD-rich cannabis when they want or need to experience quick relief of acute conditions, such as nausea, anxiety, certain types of pain, or migraines. The near-immediate onset also allows you to adjust and find a desired dose, since you don't have to wait long to see if what you just inhaled is working. For those new to THC-rich cannabis, overdose (getting too high) is relatively short-lived when inhaling compared to other methods.

You can choose to smoke a CBD-rich cannabis preroll, or you can roll your own CBD-rich flowers. Or, if you prefer a more discreet method of consuming cannabis that avoids smelling like you just smoked a joint, you can try vaping.

Vaping CBD

Inhalation via vaping cannabis flower or oil is another option. Cannabis oil extracts can also be dabbed, which is similar to vaping, but done with a solid or wax-like concentrate melted by a dab pen before being inhaled. The main issue with smoking is that smoke can irritate the lungs. Although smoking cannabis is not associated with

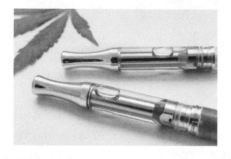

CBD vape pens

lung cancer or COPD, there are adverse health issues (chronic cough, congestion) associated with breathing any kind of smoke.

You'll feel the effects from vaping CBD slightly slower than if you smoke it, but you'll absorb more CBD.[11] Although vaping is generally less of an irritant to the lungs, thinning agents and other additives in oil extracts and cartridges can break down into carcinogens when heated in poor-quality vaporizers. This is not an issue when vaporizing organic cannabis flowers rather than an oil concentrate.

If you choose to vape, buy your vaping device from a reputable outlet, like a state-licensed dispensary. Avoid liquid CBD extracts that contain propylene glycol, polyethylene glycol, vitamin E acetate,

Transdermal CBD

Though you technically apply transdermal patches to your skin, their effects are nothing like topicals. Transdermal patches are supposed to deliver CBD through the skin and into your bloodstream for a body-wide systemic effect. A transdermal delivery vehicle is designed to release therapeutic compounds into the bloodstream at a con-

stant rate. If a CBD-rich transdermal patch also contains THC, the user may experience intoxicating effects, depending on how much THC and CBD are in the patch.

Transdermal administration should confer an experience somewhat like sublingual use, although a transdermal patch could be designed to work for longer periods of time. It's

worth noting, however, that a transdermal CBD isolate failed to treat epilepsy in a clinical trial, whereas a sublingual CBD isolate was successful.

Any company claiming to market a CBD-infused transdermal product should provide to consumers access to data demonstrating how well it is actually absorbed.

Suppositories

CBD oil–infused suppositories are a relative newcomer to the burgeoning CBD market. Think of these products as topicals that are applied internally by insertion either rectally or vaginally. Rectal and vaginal suppositories have both been used to deliver medicine to people in many cultures around the world for centuries. Vaginal application impacts the pelvic region, which houses a matrix of nerves that travel to the legs and up the spine; and the colon contains cannabinoid receptors CB_1 and CB_2.[12]

Rectal administration of cannabis oil may activate the cannabinoid receptors located there. The rectum also contains a number of key veins that deliver blood to the entire body, but it doesn't appear that suppositories facilitate much cannabinoid absorption into the bloodstream.

Anecdotally, men and women have reported using rectal suppositories to treat anal fissures, hemorrhoid inflammation, digestive issues, Crohn's and IBS, sciatica, restless leg syndrome, lower back pain, prostate issues, cancer, and postoperative pain.

Women have reported using vaginal suppositories to ease menstrual cramps, abdominal pain, endometriosis, pelvic discomfort, postcoital pain or inflammation, vaginal dryness, and pain with intercourse, as well as for relaxation and sexual enhancement.

Although many anecdotal reports are positive, the science is far from conclusive. A lot more research is needed to better understand exactly how this method of using CBD works (or doesn't).[13]

flavorings, or other dubious additives. As of Februrary 2020, more than 2,800 people had been hospitalized and 68 people had died during an outbreak of vaping-related lung injury; many of these cases were associated with vaping contaminated cannabis oil.[14]

Topicals

You don't have to smoke or ingest CBD to enjoy its benefits. You also can apply it topically. CBD-infused lotions, rubs, and/or balms that you apply directly to your skin over an inflamed area are popular for muscle aches and joint soreness from conditions like arthritis as well as certain skin conditions. Many topical CBD lotions and balms also contain common over-the-counter ingredients such as menthol, lidocaine, capsaicin, or camphor, making it difficult to determine if a positive effect is due to the CBD, another ingredient, or a combination thereof. The strength of product you need depends on the level of discomfort you're experiencing along with how you personally respond to CBD.

Onset: Seconds to minutes.

Dose: Not well-established.

Distribution: Locally; it affects the area to which it is applied.

Duration: Several hours. Variable, depending on other components in the topical product.

When applied topically, CBD and THC do not enter your bloodstream directly; rather they interact with cannabinoid receptors throughout the epidermis. Certain cannabis terpenes, such as limonene or nerolidol (also known as penetrol), can help CBD and THC permeate the skin locally, but not enough to get it into the blood systemically. But terpenes are tricky compounds; too large a concentration of terpenes in a topical product may irritate and damage the skin.

While salves and creams may be beneficial for certain conditions, the verdict is still out as to whether CBD bath bombs, which dissolve in a tub of hot water, are effective as a therapy, other than the fact that soaking in a hot bath is mentally and physically relaxing.

Buyer Beware: CBD-Infused Products

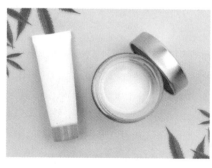
CBD creams and lotions

With current market predictions estimating CBD sales at over $20 billion in the United States alone, it's no wonder other business sectors want to get in on the act. The food and beverage market came on board, as did cosmetics and beauty. Now companies are hawking supposed CBD-infused clothing, mattresses, pillows, and even hair products. All of this has industry insiders scratching their heads.

Chances are you're every bit as confused. Here's a rundown of all the odd places you may be seeing CBD infusion, and you can decide whether any of it is worth your money.[15]

CBD Activewear: Taking CBD oil before or after a workout is a fitness trend of the moment. Whether it actually speeds recovery between training sessions has yet to be proven in a lab, but many in the active sports community swear by it.

"I Tried It"

Alex Malkin, 39, San Diego, California

For 10 years, Alex Malkin would wake up every day at around 4 a.m. unable to sleep. After trying many medications to help his insomnia, he found that only drugs like SleepAid would work, but they left him feeling groggy every morning after a near-sleepless night. "It was harder to work in this state than after a sleepless night."

One day, he began using CBD at the advice of a friend. The results changed everything; the sleepless nights were no longer. "Three days later, a real miracle happened," Malkin said. "I was sleeping all night without waking up. I was shocked! It has changed my life for the better." Malkin has continued taking a CBD tincture and has felt his sleep improve dramatically since.

Since he works on a computer all day, Malkin's neck and back are usually hurting and stiff. "I used to use painkillers, chemical creams, and ibuprofen; but now I completely abandoned them because of creams containing CBD,

which have fast absorption and help with the same efficiency," he said. Now, he no longer needs to use sleep medication to get to sleep and stay asleep. After suffering from insomnia for a decade, he's now able to stay asleep all night and wake rested instead of tired and groggy.

"Honestly, now I take CBD only two to three times a week because my sleep has already returned to normal," Malkin said. "The vape gives the fastest effect, but the impact of it passes as fast as it appeared. It is suitable for relieving stress after a working day, but for a good sleep, oil and gummies are more useful for me."

Some manufacturers have exploited the CBD fitness trend to market products like CBD-infused activewear, which may seem fashionable but is without any beneficial function.

These products, such as CBD-infused leggings, jumpsuits, and sports bras claim that skin friction and muscle movement cause CBD to be released so it then can be absorbed through the skin.

There is no evidence to substantiate those claims; and given how poorly CBD is absorbed into the skin, the odds of clothes being able to deliver therapeutic amounts are slim to zero.

CBD Hair and Beauty Products: Research shows that CBD's anti-inflammatory and immunoregulating action can penetrate through the skin when delivered by a specially formulated cream.[16] So it's not a stretch of the imagination to consider that CBD might make a worthy therapeutic addition to skincare products for inflamed or difficult-to-treat skin conditions like acne or psoriasis.

However, when it comes to adding CBD for hair products, the evidence-based jury is definitely out. In the case where CBD products are designed to calm an irritated scalp, logic might suggest that CBD could be of benefit. But CBD beard oil or CBD hair detangler? There's no sound thinking—or science—there.

CBD-Infused Pillows and Mattresses: You can buy CBD-infused pillows and mattresses that reportedly work the same way as the athletic wear: Droplets of CBD are bonded to the pillow or mattress surface. The friction of your skin and hair gently breaks the microcapsules and releases CBD so you get "microdoses" during the night for sustained rest.

If you need a new mattress or pillow and you like these products, they likely can't hurt you, but there's absolutely no evidence that miniscule doses delivered through contact with fabric will help you, either. There are far better ways to try the supplement than CBD-impregnated pillows (especially at $129 each).

8

Buying CBD

I
T'S NOT AN exaggeration to say that you can buy CBD pretty much everywhere these days. Gas stations, grocery stores, big box stores, convenience markets, and countless online outlets are selling CBD, as well as licensed dispensaries in states where cannabis is legal for medical or adult use.

Unfortunately, there is little regulatory oversight for manufacturing and selling hemp-derived CBD products, which can lead to confusion at best and outright deception at worst. Many hemp-derived products are mislabeled as to CBD and THC content. One study (among several with similar findings) published in the *Journal of the American Medical Association* reported that 69 percent of 85 product samples bought over the Internet did not have the amount of CBD and/or THC shown on the label.[17]

Another review found that some hemp-derived CBD brands falsely claim full-spectrum CBD-rich oil is in their products when lab tests of several samples revealed only one cannabinoid—CBD—was present, indicating that these products were made with a CBD isolate rather than a whole-plant CBD-rich extract.[18]

Another problem: Some hemp-derived CBD products may be tainted with toxic solvent residues, because the plants are like sponges for heavy metals, pesticides, and potentially harmful chemicals that may be in the soil or water where they're grown. Still others are overly processed with thinning agents, corn syrup, artificial flavors and colors, and other additives and toxins.

In short, there's a lot of snake oil along with high-quality CBD on the market right now. So, it's important to be able to tell the difference, find a trusted source, know what you're buying, and know what form to buy it in.

Where to Shop

First and foremost, skip the gas station/convenience store point-of-purchase stuff. You want to find the most trustworthy, reputable source possible for your CBD products. The best place to start depends on where you live. If you live in a state where medical marijuana is legal, get your CBD products from a state-licensed dispensary, where the products have been rigorously tested for cannabinoid content, pesticide, and solvent residues and the staff should include educated cannabis consultants who can walk you through the product selection.

If you don't reside in a state or country with legal cannabis dispensaries, you can access CBD products via online storefronts or from actual CBD brick-and-mortar stores. The more information provided by your CBD source, the better.

As mentioned on page 145, you'll be choosing from a variety of product types. They are not all readily available to everyone because of differences in state and federal laws.

Some states still restrict CBD purchase and possession to only those with a prescription. In Idaho and Kansas, it is illegal to buy a CBD product that contains any THC, even if it's less than 0.3 percent. In other states, the laws are extremely murky, leaving consumers and shopkeepers to fend for themselves in interpreting them. (Examine the map on page 16 to see what's currently legal in your state.) Here's what to consider depending upon the product type you're looking for.

Pharmaceutical CBD. As the name indicates, pharmaceutical CBD is just that—CBD that you pick up with a prescription at your pharmacy. Only those who are prescribed Epidiolex have the option of buying pharmaceutical CBD. Some CBD products are touted as "pharmaceutical grade" but are not actually FDA-approved pharmaceuticals.

CBD isolates and/or broad-spectrum CBD concentrates (with no THC). You can find unregulated CBD isolate and THC-free broad-spectrum products in all 50 states. If you live in a state that has restrictive cannabis and/or CBD laws and you want to buy a CBD isolate, visit a CBD specialty store where you can ask questions and get information about specific products. If there are no CBD stores in your region, an online retailer that provides detailed product information is likely your best option.

> Some states still restrict CBD purchase and possession to only those with a prescription.

Full-spectrum hemp-derived CBD (less than 0.3 percent THC). Hemp-derived CBD products with less than 0.3 percent THC are seemingly legal on the federal level (though this is still a bit of a gray zone because the FDA is not regulating these products) but are still illegal under some state laws that prohibit any amount of THC.

Full-spectrum cannabis-derived CBD with more than 0.3 percent THC. These products fall under the label of medical marijuana because they exceed the 0.3 percent THC limit that defines hemp. Dispensaries in states that have legalized cannabis for therapeutic and/or recreational use may sell a variety of CBD-rich products high in CBD and relatively low in THC.

CBD-rich cannabis with a significant amount of THC. These products are also considered to be medical marijuana because they exceed the 0.3 percent THC limit that defines hemp. Dispensaries in states that have legalized marijuana for therapeutic and/or recreational use may sell a variety of balanced cannabis products that contain roughly equal amounts of CBD and THC or substantial amounts of both.

What to Buy

When considering a hemp-based CBD product for therapeutic or wellness purposes, Project CBD generally recommends choosing full-spectrum CBD oil extracts rather than isolates or products labeled "pure CBD" or "no THC." As the name implies, full spectrum means the product includes the essential oil extracted from hemp or cannabis with all the naturally occurring compounds, including a small amount of THC, so you can get the synergistic benefit of the entourage effect and the best medicinal value.

If you are buying CBD-rich cannabis products from a licensed dispensary, you will find that they come in a variety of ratios of CBD to THC. Ratios can range from 1:1 (equal amounts CBD to THC) to 40:1, which will have 40 times more CBD than THC.

If THC is completely illegal in your state or if you're concerned about getting drug tested for THC, consider opting for broad-spectrum CBD oil products, which are supposed to have the THC removed. You'll still get some of the benefits of the other cannabis compounds without worrying about the legality or presence of THC in your system.

What to Look for

Being an informed CBD consumer is a must if you want to buy a quality product free of contaminants and that actually contains what it says on the label. It helps to know the source of the CBD, where it comes from and how it was extracted, but this information isn't always readily available.

Prior to the 2018 Farm Bill, many if not most of the CBD products available in the United States were derived from low-resin industrial hemp grown in Europe and China. It's better to purchase products

How to Read a Label

As you might imagine, there are no standardized labels for CBD products. But at a minimum, there should be some indication of the form of CBD you're buying (full-spectrum, broad-spectrum, or isolate), how much CBD is in the product, and what else, if anything, is in the bottle. Here's what to look for:

❶ Milligrams of CBD: Every product should clearly state how many milligrams (mg) are in the entire package.

❷ Serving size: How much of the product is considered one serving (e.g., 20 drops of a tincture, 1 gummy).

Dose: How many milligrams of CBD you get per one serving.

❸ Number of servings per package: How many doses you will get out of a product (e.g., 30 servings/600 drops of tincture, 30 gummies).

Potency/strength/ concentration: Potency refers to how much of a given substance is needed to have an effect. The

higher the concentration, the more potent the product is and the more CBD you'll get per serving. See page 175 for more on CBD potency and concentrations.

❹ Other ingredients: The label should list all relevant ingredients, including THC and other cannabinoids, and additives such as coloring and flavoring additives, preservatives, and texturizing agents. A full ingredient list should also include carrier oils like glycerin and propylene glycol. When buying CBD vape pens, avoid thinners, thickeners, vitamins, and flavoring additives. Beware of terms like "natural ingredients," which can include problematic additives like vegetable oil, which is generally not a good thing to inhale into your lungs.

Recommended use: The label should clearly tell you how to use the product, though it may not tell you specific dosing directions. (See Chapter 9 for dosing instructions.)

Disclaimers: Expect to see disclaimers that the Food and Drug Administration has not evaluated the product.

QR code: Some states require and many products include a QR (quick response) code on the label that you can scan for batch info; it includes COA (certificate of analysis) data and other relevant information regarding the purity and quality of the product, extraction date, and analysis date. QR codes are a sign of quality.

Third-party certification: A stamp indicating third-party certification attests to the accuracy of the label. This information may also be part of the COA.

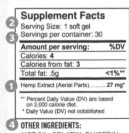

made from high-resin CBD-rich plants with a robust terpene profile, the kind now being grown in various parts of the United States. If you're buying from a dispensary or a retail store, ask the staff where the CBD in their products are sourced. They may not always know.

Consumer Reports suggests looking for products made by companies in U.S. states that have legalized the recreational and medical use of cannabis, since they tend to have stricter regulatory standards. If you live in a "CBD-only" state, choose CBD products made with American-grown hemp (a rapidly expanding list that includes Colorado, Kentucky, Oregon, Montana, Vermont, Tennessee, and New York, among others). If possible, seek out CBD products derived from cannabis grown sustainably in accordance with organic standards to avoid harmful pesticide residues.

These are some factors that make a CBD brand stand out amid a crowded marketplace:

- CBD brands that manufacture products with the full spectrum of cannabis/hemp components, including THC.
- Brands that don't minimize or trivialize the therapeutic value of THC or the synergistic interplay between CBD and THC and other components of cannabis.
- CBD and cannabis brands that don't include the following additives in their CBD oil products: thinning agents, such as polyethylene glycol 400 (PEG 400), propylene glycol (PG); flavoring agents, especially cinnamon-, cream-, and vanilla-flavored additives; as well as corn syrup and artificial sweeteners like sucralose.
- CBD brands rigorously tested for solvent and pesticide residues.
- CBD brands that make products from hemp or cannabis grown in accordance with regenerative agricultural practices, which improve soil quality and promote carbon sequestration, which helps remove carbon dioxide from the atmosphere to reduce global climate change.

"I Tried It"

Josh Kincaid, 42,
Seattle, Washington

When Josh Kincaid, 42, set out to climb all 832 steps of the Space Needle in downtown Seattle for a charity race, he worried that he might not be able to complete the journey due to the severe neck and back pain he had suffered since a job injury more than 20 years earlier. But thanks to a transdermal CBD patch, he was able to complete it without a problem.

"I don't think I could have done the stair climb without CBD," Kincaid said. "After taking CBD, I no longer have to take opioids or muscle relaxants for chronic pain nor the antinausea medication to stop the 8-hour-long nausea I used to get from migraines."

Kincaid first tried CBD after he left a stressful job as a financial analyst to start a cannabis café. Inspired by his high school friend, who had begun to use medical marijuana to treat his multiple sclerosis (MS), the café served a coffee infused with CBD and THC. Kincaid realized that CBD not only helped ease his physical pain but also helped him overcome the extreme anxiety that used to prevent him from any public speaking. Now, he runs a podcast about the business of cannabis and hemp. Kincaid also credits CBD with helping him deal with cravings when he changed his diet and lost a third of his body weight.

CBD can be digested in a dizzying array of differ-ent forms, from gummies to creams to tinctures taken under the tongue. "It took me years to figure out the best delivery methods and doses," Kincaid said. "I use a topical cream for neck pain. While on the go or for immediate relief, I use a vape pen because the effect is incredibly quick. Edibles last longer, so they're great for sleep. At home I use a tincture and 'stack' it 24 hours prior to a big event."

"People are coming to me because I look so healthy now," Kincaid marveled. "My wife takes CBD when her ulcerative colitis flares up. My mom is asking about CBD. I even gave my dog CBD when she had cancer— you could literally feel the heat dissipate from her tumor and see the wrinkles on her forehead relax after each dose."

Choose Products That List Amount per Serving: Look for products that tell you how much CBD and/or THC you're getting per serving, not just the total cannabinoid content in the entire bottle. This can help you avoid dosing confusion, and it's also extra assurance that what you're buying actually contains the ingredients you're looking for. When shopping online, don't be afraid to contact CBD companies directly and ask questions. And if you cannot reach them directly, try another brand.

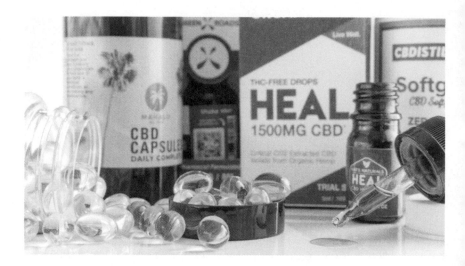

Some products will label themselves as "whole-plant" or "full-spectrum" and may even list a total amount of "cannabinoids" but will not list CBD amounts on the label. This could be a red flag that you are buying a low-quality, resin-deficient hemp product that contains little or maybe even zero CBD. Or it could just mean that the company has opted not to list the CBD amount as a tactic to sidestep FDA scrutiny. If you're at all unsure what's in a bottle you're looking to buy, check the COA. If you can't find the answer to your question, ask the company. If you cannot reach the company or they can't give you an answer, consider choosing a different brand.

Beware Outlandish Claims: If a manufacturer promises to cure anything, be wary. If a manufacturer makes explicit health claims, that's a red flag. Making health claims is legal only for prescription drugs and is strictly forbidden by the FDA and the Federal Trade Commission when it comes to supplements like CBD products. The FDA has sporadically cracked down on CBD manufacturers that make prohibited health claims. But it's like playing federal whack-a-mole; as soon as a warning is issued, other brands make the same mistake. Avoid these products.

Avoid Additive-Laden Edibles: You're buying CBD products to improve your health, so be sure the products you choose fall in line with your general standards for buying high-quality foods. Avoid CBD-infused gummies or edibles that contain corn syrup and artificial colors, as well as those laden with added sweeteners (to mask the somewhat bitter flavor of CBD oil extracts). Read your labels. If a CBD product contains additives you wouldn't want in the food you put on your table, don't accept the same additives in the supplements you ingest.

Beware Marketing Scams: The Internet is full of online retailers looking to exploit consumers. You should be able to buy a single CBD product without signing up for any sort of membership or recurring purchases. If the purchasing process seems overly complicated, requires you to sign up for a subscription or membership service, or makes you buy more than you want, consider looking elsewhere for your CBD products.

Be Prepared to Pay for Quality: There's no getting around it: CBD products aren't cheap. Many factors contribute to this, including the ambiguous legal environment pertaining to hemp and cannabis, which increases the risks and costs for manufacturers. It's hard to pin down an exact price range for CBD products, but expect to pay for quality.

Check the Certificate of Analysis (COA): Legalities and technicalities aside, hemp-derived CBD is just a mouse click or a phone tap away for anyone willing to roll the dice and purchase CBD oil products that are manufactured with little regulatory oversight. You want to look for a product that has gone through independent lab testing for quality assurance.

A CBD manufacturer should be able to produce a third-party certificate of analysis (COA) that shows how their products performed on screenings for CBD, THC, and any contaminants. California's medical cannabis regulations require CBD products to

How to Store Your CBD

Like many medications, CBD products keep best if you store them in a cool, dark place, as heat and direct sunlight can cause them to degrade. That means if you live in a hot climate without air conditioning, you should keep your CBD in the refrigerator. CBD also degrades when it's exposed to air, so keep the packaging tightly sealed. Properly stowed and stored, CBD should maintain its effectiveness for about a year or even longer.

be tested by an independent third-party-accredited laboratory and may fine distributors if they are found to have falsified COA data. Some states also require—and many manufacturers provide—a QR code on the label of CBD products, so you can download their COA to your mobile device and inspect it before you try or buy.

A COA should include the product batch number; CBD and THC levels (not just the total amount of plant cannabinoids); and certification indicating that heavy metals, pesticides, and solvent residues fall within the range of allowable limits. In most states, however, allowable limits have not been established, and there is a lack of consistency among states where allowable limits have been established.

Keep in mind that a COA is only as meaningful as the regulatory framework in which it's generated. In an unregulated or poorly regulated environment, for instance, a lab can charge extra money for providing the results that the manufacturer is seeking. And it would be difficult for a consumer to know if the COA is accurate and/or if it actually corresponds to the batch number of a particular product. Be that as it may, if a COA is available, it's definitely worth comparing what it says about a product with what's on the product label.

9

Dosing CBD

M EDICINE ONLY DOES its job correctly if you take it correctly. So, if you're using CBD medicinally, proper dosing is key. Unfortunately, that's not always easy to nail down with precision.

Like so much involving CBD, figuring out the right dose can take some time and effort. Unlike a bottle of Advil that provides detailed dosing directions right on the label, many CBD brands leave that up to you. CBD manufacturers will generally list how much of the product is considered to be a single serving, but how many servings you need to take to see results for any particular condition is not specified. Nor should it be. Because only one CBD product has been approved by the FDA (Epidiolex), other CBD products are not allowed to make medical claims.

The amount of CBD needed to feel an effect also varies from person to person and condition to condition. Multiple factors influence how you'll respond to CBD, including your gender (estrogen interacts with the endocannabinoid system, which can influence its effect), your age (drug metabolism in general decreases with age), your weight, and the health of your endocannabinoid system.

Your DNA also plays a role. Just as people have different tolerances to substances like alcohol or other medications, individuals react differently to CBD. Your personal genetics strongly influence your CYP enzyme (the family of enzymes that break down drugs and other substances in your liver) activity, which is responsible for CBD metabolism. In fact, according to a study published in *Frontiers in Genetics*, activity of CYP3A4—the most important drug-metabolizing enzyme in humans—can vary more than 100-fold from person to person, and genetics accounts for the nearly 90 percent of that variability.[19] If you are someone who metabolizes CBD more slowly, you will likely experience an extended effect after taking a dose. If you are a fast metabolizer, you may need a larger dose for desired effects. To find out if you metabolize CBD quickly or slowly, you will need to use some trial and error.

Also, as you'll recall, high and low doses of CBD can sometimes produce opposite effects. Being able to start low, go slow, and control the dosing can make it easier to figure out the right dose for you.

You'll also experience different effects depending on what type of CBD product you're using and how you're consuming it. For example, a 2015 Israeli study concluded that full-spectrum CBD-rich cannabis oil is effective at much lower doses and has a wider therapeutic window, meaning it is effective in a wider range of doses, than a CBD isolate. "The therapeutic synergy observed with plant extracts results in the requirement for a lower amount of active components, with consequent reduced adverse side effects," concluded the researchers.[20] CBD isolates, on the other hand, require very high—and precise—doses to be effective, according to animal studies. Problematic drug interactions are also more likely with a high-dose CBD isolate than with whole-plant cannabis essential oil.

Products like vaping oils and tinctures, which don't need to go through digestion and liver metabolism, often work faster and require lower doses than capsules and edibles. With all of these variables, it can be challenging even for trained professionals to dial in dosing.

"Dosing cannabis is unlike any therapeutic agent to which I was exposed in my medical training," says Dustin Sulak, DO, the director of Integr8 Health, in Maine. "Some patients effectively use tiny amounts of cannabis, while others use incredibly high doses. I've seen adult patients achieve therapeutic effects at 1 mg of total cannabinoids daily, while others consume over 2,000 mg daily without adverse effects."

CBD studies echo and affirm Sulak's experience. CBD doses administered in human trials are all over the map, ranging from 5 mg CBD to 600 mg or more. Again, be prepared to experiment and take notes as you start using CBD.

Getting Started with CBD

The general rule of thumb for dosing with cannabis-based products (including CBD products) is to "start low and go slow." In other words, begin with a low dose and gradually increase the amount as needed or until you start to experience diminished or adverse effects. It's wise to follow the same rule of thumb for hemp-based CBD products with little or no THC.

In some cases, physicians who specialize in cannabis medicine may recommend that a first-time CBD user start with a single serving—just one drop or one gel cap. This helps ensure that you don't have any adverse reactions to the product. Adverse reactions are uncommon, but it's possible to be allergic to a CBD product that may include additives, which can cause problematic reactions. So start with just one or two drops of tinctures, a single puff of vapor, or a small bite of an edible, and give yourself time—an hour or more for tinctures or edibles and a few minutes for vaporizer products—to see if you feel any ill effects like itching, hives, heartburn, sneezing, or diarrhea. Serious allergic side effects are extremely rare, but call your doctor if you experience any strong adverse reactions such as swelling, difficulty breathing, or vomiting.

Once you've established that you haven't had an adverse reaction

What the Research Says

Research on using CBD therapeutically is in its infancy. But some scientists and doctors have been trying to get a handle on how much of the cannabinoid is needed to have beneficial effects for various conditions.

In one study titled "Cannabidiol in Humans— The Quest for Therapeutic Targets," researchers combed through existing literature to come up with a few answers. They found doses of oral CBD isolate in the range of 150 mg to 600 mg a day may have a beneficial effect on social anxiety disorder, insomnia, and epilepsy.[21] And research on general sleep disorders has shown benefits with a wide range of doses.

For movement disorders, like Parkinson's and Huntington's disease, researchers found the most success with doses in the range of 10 mg of CBD isolate per kg of body weight. For a 150-pound (68 kg) adult, that would translate to 680 mg a day.[22]

For chronic pain, clinical studies involving Sativex, a pharmaceutical sublingual tincture with nearly equal amounts of CBD and THC, indicate the op-timal dosage to be 21 mg a day; whereas patients who received twice that dose experienced some pain relief, but it wasn't as effective as the smaller dose. And when the dose of Sativex was doubled again to 84 mg per day, it had no painkilling effect at all. Don't assume that a CBD isolate or a broad-spectrum product without THC will be just as effective at 21 mg a day as Sativex, which includes a significant amount of THC. There's no clinical research showing that a 21 mg of CBD isolate will have a notable painkilling effect.[23]

It's difficult at this time to say how much CBD might be too much. According to a review published in Mayo Clinic Proceedings titled "Clinician's Guide to Cannabidiol and Hemp Oils," CBD doses of up to 300 mg per day have been used safely for up to six months, and doses of 1,200 mg to 1,500 mg per day were safely used for up to four weeks. In studies on Epidiolex (the CBD treatment prescribed for people with three types of epilepsy), these large, therapeutic doses caused adverse side effects like sleepiness, decreased appetite, and diarrhea in about a third of patients. But these side effects were not necessarily due to the CBD per se; they could be attributable to additives like sucralose and ethanol that are present in Epidiolex. Be that as it may, the side effects triggered by Epidiolex were less severe and less frequent than the harsh side effects associated with other pharmaceutical medications for pediatric epilepsy.[24]

Most people who use CBD for sleep, anxiety, or other everyday health issues are taking much smaller doses than those administered in extensive preclinical and limited clinical studies. In part, that's because most of the studies utilize CBD isolates rather than full- or broad-spectrum CBD. Also, many of these studies are looking at more serious diseases and conditions. If you suffer from such a condition, it's especially important to work with your doctor if you plan to take CBD, especially high doses, on a regular basis.

to the product, begin with a reasonable minimal dose of 5 mg to 10 mg of active ingredient. If you're satisfied there, stop. If not, increase the dose slightly every other day or two until you start to experience benefits. If you start to feel worse or have negative symptoms like fatigue, dial back the dosage.

If you are ingesting CBD, take it with food (especially healthy fats) or after a meal—except if you are administering a CBD tincture sublingually (in which case you want to avoid swallowing it). Animal research shows that oral CBD absorption and bioavailability increase three- to six-fold when taken with food compared to on an empty stomach.[25] Research on people has duplicated these findings. Scientists at GW Pharmaceuticals, which develops cannabis-derived pharmaceuticals (Epidiolex and Sativex), found that administering CBD (in this case a large dose of 750 mg) after a light 400-calorie breakfast tripled CBD absorption, and a heavy 900-calorie breakfast quadrupled it.[26]

Before you start taking any supplements, it's generally a good idea to check in with your doctor. Unfortunately, not many physicians are well versed in CBD's health effects, and there are few gold-standard double-blind studies on human subjects for doctors to reference. That being said, any physician with an open mind should be able to help you figure out if you're using medications that may interact with CBD. (See page 185 for more on drug interactions.)

Dosing Different Ways of Taking CBD

Because different methods of taking CBD enter your bloodstream and/or interact with your endocannabinoid system through different avenues, each delivery system may require a different approach to dosing. Here are some tips for developing a dosing regimen that's appropriate for the four main ways of administering CBD: oral, sublingual, inhalation, and topical.

Oral Ingestion: Edible CBD products are easy to use and understand. The label should clearly state how much CBD is in each dose of what you're eating or drinking or the supplement you're swallowing. If you want to take 25 mg of CBD, you can simply take a 25 mg capsule and you're done.

Taking CBD with food—or as part of a food—can slow digestion but ultimately may improve your body's ability to absorb CBD. For the best effect, take CBD with some healthy fats (walnuts, salmon, avocado, coconut, etc.). Research shows that consuming CBD, which is fat-soluble, with fats increases the amount of CBD that passes through the digestive tract and can almost triple the amount of CBD that reaches your bloodstream. Researchers have also found that certain supplements may help boost CBD absorption. In one study on rodents, piperine, a compound found in black pepper, increased the maximum concentration of CBD in the bloodstream six-fold compared to a supplement without piperine, by helping transport the cannabinoid across the intestine and blocking the enzymes that break it down. But those studies have not been done in humans.[27]

Though it takes longer—generally between one to two hours—to take effect, orally ingested CBD may have the longest lasting impact (four or more hours), since an orally consumed CBD molecule stays in the body longer than it does through other methods.

Sublingual Administration: Because it bypasses your digestive system, taking CBD sublingually (that is, placing it under your tongue) is one of the quickest and most effective ways to get CBD into your bloodstream. The relative quick action of sublingual tinctures makes them a good choice for pain, anxiety, and sleep. The key here is holding the oil under your tongue for a minute or more before swallowing (otherwise, you may as well just take CBD in an edible/capsule form). You may be able to get even more CBD out of every drop by holding it under the tongue for the recommended amount of time and then swishing it around in your mouth before swallowing to allow the oil to make contact with your cheeks and gums as well.

When using CBD drops, you'll need to meter out your dosage with the dropper. When buying tinctures, look for products that show how much CBD you get not just in the whole bottle but in each dose (spray, drop, or mL), so you're not stuck using a calculator to figure out how much you're taking per any given number of drops or per spray.

For instance, if you have a 30 mL bottle of 600 mg CBD, each dropper will contain 20 mg of CBD (600 mg/30 mL = 20 mg per mL), and each drop will contain 1 mg of CBD (20 mg/20 drops = 1). But dosing is far easier when these amounts are clearly labeled on the product.

Inhalation: The quickest way to get CBD into your system and the easiest to titrate is by inhaling it into your lungs. Not only does this method bypass digestion, but also the lungs are extremely vascular, so the molecule swiftly passes into your bloodstream and moves straight to your brain and central nervous system quickly. From there, it gets metabolized by your liver and cleared out of your body.

Smoking or vaping might be best reserved for situations where you need fast-acting relief, especially since smoking will irritate the lungs, and the long-term health effects of using various unregulated vaping devices is still not known.

Dosing with a vaporizer is relatively simple because the effects are felt so quickly. That makes it easy to titrate, or measure, adjust, and fine-tune, the dose. How much CBD you get depends on how long you inhale. Instead of inhaling a large amount of vapor into your lungs all at once, try drawing in a puff without entirely filling your lungs and then continue in the same breath by drawing a deep, full inhalation of plain air before exhaling.[28] This way you have a stream of vape-free air pushing the CBD-infused vapor past your trachea and fully into your lungs, where the exchange between your alveoli and blood circulation happens. You're not taking in more than you need, and you can better absorb each dose. The same goes for smoking. There's no need to take a huge hit of a joint and hold it for as long as possible. As soon as you inhale, the CBD will enter your bloodstream via the lungs.

If you decide to vape, avoid CBD vape cartridges made with thinning agents, or carriers such as propylene glycol, vegetable glycerin, or MCT oil. These compounds may have adverse health effects when heated and inhaled.[29]

Intranasal administration is another way to "inhale" CBD. In terms of dosing, animal studies on intranasal CBD have been promising, showing that CBD administered through a nasal mist is absorbed within 10 minutes and has high bioavailability, with between 34 percent and 46 percent of the molecule reaching the bloodstream.[30] Like other forms of CBD, nasal sprays come in different strengths or CBD potencies, such as 200 mg bottles that deliver 1 mg CBD per spray and 400 mg bottles that deliver twice that with 2 mg per spray.

For the best results, use as directed, and do not snort the spray, which will essentially send it down the back of your throat and into your stomach, where your digestive enzymes will metabolize much of the active ingredient. Instead, place the tip of the nozzle just inside your nostril; aim toward your ear (to fully mist the passages), and compress the spray plunger. Then sniff in gently, just enough to keep the mist from dripping out.

Topical and Transdermal Application: Because they confer effects via the cannabinoid receptors in your skin and don't enter the bloodstream, the bioavailability of balms, creams, salves, and rubs tends to be low. That's not to say that people do not find relief from these products.

Animal studies show that topical CBD application can help reduce

Understanding CBD Concentrations

Along with being available in full-spectrum, broad-spectrum, and/or isolate products, CBD is also sold in various strengths or concentrations. For CBD-infused tinctures, these concentrations range from 100 mg to 5,000 mg for a single bottle.

These numbers refer to the potency of the product. Potency is an expression of the activity of the drug in terms of the amount required to produce an effect. The higher the concentration, the more potent the product and the more CBD you'll get per serving. For example, a 1 mL dose (about 20 drops of oil) from a tincture of a low-potency 300 mg (30 mL) product will deliver about 10 mg of CBD. That allows you to start low, with perhaps half that amount, and see how you respond. If you dive right in with a high-potency 1,200 mg (30 mL) bottle, you're getting 40 mg of CBD for that same 1 mL dose.

You can expect to pay more for higher-potency CBD because you don't need as high of a dose and the bottle will last longer. Here's a look at what might be considered low-, moderate-, and high-potency products (based on a standard 30 mL bottle):

Low-Potency: 100 mg to 300 mg per bottle. Manufacturers generally market these products as being good for general wellness and stress relief. This is a good place to start to see if CBD is right for you.

Medium-Potency: 500 mg to 600 mg per bottle. If you find yourself taking multiple doses of a low-potency product, it makes sense to step up to a more concentrated product, such as a medium-potency CBD oil. This range is popular for general anxiety, minor sleep issues, inflammation, and daily aches and pains from exercise and/or medical conditions like arthritis.

High-Potency: 1,000 mg and above per bottle. As you'd expect, higher-potency CBD may be appropriate for more serious issues like insomnia, deep muscle soreness, migraines, and more. Generally, first-time users are not advised to start out with higher-potency products unless a physician recommends a substantial dosage regimen to treat a specific condition. Of course, you can also microdose a high-potency product, and you still may get more CBD per serving than a higher dose of a low-potency product.

When buying CBD edibles, you can generally choose from a range of concentrations—from low-potency edibles, such as 10 mg gummies, to moderately high-concentration edibles, like 50 mg gummies (or it might be possible to find some supercharged gummies that deliver 100 mg per edible, but that is not the norm).

Vape oils can range in strength from 50 mg cartridges all the way up to very high 4,000 mg cartridges.

Topical CBD products like balms and lotions are also sold in a variety of concentrations from low-concentration products in the 250 mg to 300 mg range to high-concentration products with 1,000 mg or more.

inflammation. Many people from professional athletes to weekend warriors use topical CBD to soothe sore muscles, and topical CBD preparations are popular among arthritis sufferers.

Because a topical has a local effect and doesn't enter the bloodstream systemically, a CBD-infused cream or balm will only work on the site where it's applied and won't be effective for conditions like anxiety, sleep disruptions, or GI conditions, which require activating cannabinoid receptors in the central nervous system or internal organs.

Apply a CBD topical as you would any other ointment or lotion—just enough so the product evenly coats the skin without slathering too much at once. Start with a small amount of a cannabis topical to see if you're sensitive to it. If you go to a CBD retail store, you may be able to sample a product to see if it works for you before making a purchase. Some people report quick relief with a CBD-infused topical, while others say they get no relief at all from these products. Look for products that also include permeability enhancers like ethanol, menthol, or camphor, which help CBD penetrate through the skin layers.

If you're interested in trying a transdermal patch, they work best on the base of your neck or somewhere near the shoulder joint, where there is less muscle and fat under the skin.

Good-quality CBD transdermal patches may come in a variety of doses. Animal research has found as little as 6.2 mg per day to be effective, but again, it's difficult to say how that translates to humans.[31] Patches will generally cost more than topical treatments. You can leave some patches on for up to three days. Some people with sensitive skin might experience a bit of irritation at the site of the patch.

CBD suppositories are applied internally, but they work a lot like topicals. Dosing via the vagina or rectum is not as simple as taking a puff or swallowing a pill. Even though suppositories bypass digestion and liver metabolism, they don't appear to generate high amounts of cannabinoids in the bloodstream. When using either rectal or vaginal suppositories, follow the directions on the packaging. Always remain lying down for at least 5 minutes—between 5 and 20 minutes for vaginal suppositories—to avoid having the suppository slip out. These products generally range between 50 mg and 150 mg of CBD per dose.

The Many "Phases" of CBD

It's natural to think "more equals more," that if you take a bigger dose of something, you will have a larger (though not necessarily a better) effect. But when it comes to cannabinoids, that's not necessarily the case, says Dr. Dustin Sulak. Instead, cannabinoids can have a biphasic effect, which is to say that the dose response curve is not straightforward.

For example, you might start taking CBD at one dose and have a response. Then you might take a little more and have a greater response. But the next time you increase your dose, your response might go down and then go down even further with an even higher dose, he says. "So, we have this bell-shaped curve. And it's that optimal dose that I'm talking about, which is right in the center, the peak of that curve, and once you go more, you're actually going to get less of a response. That's what biphasic means."[32]

Cannabinoids also can have triphasic or even multiphasic effects, Sulak says. "We see that it can go up and down and up and down. Each direction is a phase. So, if I start subtherapeutic and someone gets a benefit, that's one phase. If they go up higher and they lose benefit, that's another phase. But then often, when they really crank the dose up high, that benefit will return. Sometimes when it returns, it returns with side effects or the benefits may be a little bit different than they were at the low doses. And there's probably a phase at ultra-low doses, where people can take such a small amount and get benefit down there as well."

The dose you need may also change over time. Those who use a lot of THC regularly may develop a tolerance to it, so they'll need more of it to get an adequate effect. This may also happen with CBD in some cases. Research on people who use CBD for epilepsy indicates that about one-third of them developed a tolerance to it.[33]

According to other studies, it's possible that one can even develop what is known as a *reverse tolerance* to it: As your body adjusts and your overall health improves, you may need to take less CBD to meet your need.[34]

That's why it's a good idea to keep track of how much CBD you take. Once you've found a dose that works for you, keep track of how you feel. If that nagging pain returns or your anxiety starts to creep up, you can try increasing your dose a bit (keeping in mind that it's possible to have less efficacy once you cross your sweet spot). You can also try taking a CBD break. Research shows that even just a couple of days away from cannabinoids can help your receptors to reset and make you more sensitive to the supplements again.[35]

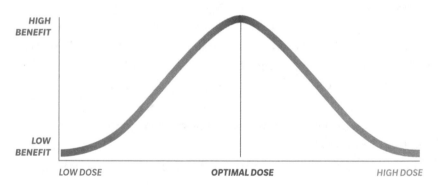

Biphasic effect

Dosing Guidelines

Finding the right dose of CBD can be a complicated process. Project CBD recommends some simple guidelines to keep in mind as you experiment with what works best for you:

1. There is no "one-size-fits-all" dose. Many factors, including age, weight, gender, and genetics, as well as the conditions you're taking

178

CBD for and the delivery method you use, all influence how much you need to feel a benefit. Be prepared to experiment.

2. Consuming CBD with food improves absorption. Animal research shows that CBD absorption and bioavailability increase three- to six-fold when taken with food compared to taken on an empty stomach. Include a little healthy fat for the best results.

3. CBD isolates require high and precise doses to be effective. CBD works best and can be used effectively in a wider range (including lower doses) when taken along with other naturally occurring cannabinoids (especially THC) and terpenes in the cannabis plant rather than as an isolated molecule.

4. CBD is safe even at high doses. According to a review published in Mayo Clinic Proceedings titled "Clinician's Guide to Cannabidiol and Hemp Oils," CBD doses of up to 300 mg per day have been used safely for up to six months, and doses of 1,200 mg to 1,500 mg per day were safely used for up to four weeks.[36]

5. Less is often more. While CBD has no serious adverse effects at any dose, an excessive amount of CBD may be less effective therapeutically than a moderate dose. And very high doses of a CBD isolate may interact with other drugs.

6. Humans are not lab rats. Don't devise a dosage regimen based on data from preclinical animal studies, which usually involve high doses of single-molecule CBD. Human metabolism differs from mice and rats, and data from animal models doesn't always translate to human experience.

7. Consider time of day. If you are in a state where medical cannabis is legal, optimizing use of CBD may entail using products with different CBD:THC ratios at different times of the day—more CBD for daylight hours, more THC at night.

8. Preventive dosing. Prolonged low-dose therapy may be advantageous for promoting wellness and staying healthy or preventing disease development or recurrence. Preclinical studies indicate that

"I Tried It"

Patricia McMillan, 74,
Phoenix, Arizona

After struggling with back problems, including sciatica, arthritis, scoliosis, and spinal stenosis, for the better of a decade, Patricia McMillan finally found relief in the form of CBD gummies.

"December 2018 was a turning point in my search for pain relief from long-time lumbar spine pain," McMillan said. "Through friends and Web research, I discovered CBD products."

McMillan started with broad-spectrum gummies with a potency of 1,500 mg, taking two gummies a day. Most of her pain resolved without any side effects. Even better, her anxiety surrounding the pain subsided.

"I had a lot of anxiety about the pain, which was much less after taking

CBD. My blood pressure also came down," McMillan said. After about three months, however, McMillan felt she was becoming habituated to the CBD.

"At some point, I was no longer getting the relief, so I moved to 5,000 mg CBD oil and used 7 drops per day," McMillan said. "This was wonderful. I felt I had finally found the right product and dosage."

Unfortunately, history repeated itself, and after another three months, McMillan found herself in-

cannabinoids have neuroprotective and cardioprotective properties that could limit the damage of a stroke or a heart attack.

9. Avoid calculating CBD dosage for an adult based on dosing pharmaceutical CBD for children. Kids and adults metabolize drugs differently. It may seem counterintuitive, but young children can tolerate high doses of cannabis oil concentrates, including THC-rich formulations, which might be daunting for an adult. Thus, it's not a good idea to calculate dosage for an adult based on what works for a child. If 1 mg/kg of CBD is an appropriate starting dose for a child, and an adult weighs 15 times more than the child, one should not assume that the correct CBD starting dose for the grownup is 15 mg/kg of body weight. That could be an excessive dose.

10. Manage psychoactivity. If you are using CBD-rich cannabis with a significant amount of THC, it's all about managing THC's tricky psychoactivity. CBD, unlike THC, is not intoxicating and can lessen or neutralize the euphoric (or dysphoric) effects of THC, creasing her dosage to get the same measure of relief.

"Again, I enjoyed great relief for a while," she said. "But the same thing would happen where the effects would wear off." She kept increasing incrementally until eventually it became prohibitively expensive to continue increasing the amount of CBD she was taking. She also was concerned about taking very high amounts indefinitely.

"I eventually reset by not taking any CBD for two months," McMillan said. "After my reset, I have been taking 1,000 mg of 1XCBD tincture under the tongue, 5 drops per day based on a dosage chart that accompanied the product. It works very fast. I have been using it for about three or four months, hoping that higher milligrams won't eventually be required."

If she runs into the same situation where she is habituated to the dose, McMillan says she'll continue to explore options, which, after getting her medical marijuana card include a CBD/THC tincture as well as doing another reset if necessary.

McMillan finds the trial and error frustrating but is grateful for the pain relief and some of the unexpected benefits of CBD. "One unforeseen benefit is that I no longer have terrible white coat syndrome," she said. "I would always be in a real state when I had to see a doctor. It was bad. I'm much less anxious now."

depending on how much of each compound is in a given product. In essence, the goal with medical cannabis is to take a CBD-rich product with as much THC as one is comfortable with. The more THC in a CBD-rich product, the more effective that product will likely be for many (but not all) conditions.

11. Don't be afraid to experiment. If you're new to CBD or cannabis medicine or if you're seeking to improve your therapeutic routine, remember this advice from Dr. Sulak: "Start low, go slow, and don't be afraid to go all the way!"

CBD Safety

A

S CBD CONTINUES to grow in popularity, many people are wondering, "Is it really safe?"

The World Health Organization (WHO) thinks so. In 2018, their Expert Committee on Drug Dependence issued a critical review report on CBD, which concluded:

> *"CBD is generally well tolerated with a good safety profile...[and] exhibits no effects indicative of any abuse or dependence potential. Reported adverse effects may be as a result of drug–drug interactions between CBD and patients' existing medications. Several countries have modified their national controls to accommodate CBD as a medicinal product. To date, there is no evidence of recreational use of CBD or any public health–related problems associated with the use of pure CBD."*[37]

The Federal Drug Administration, however, has not responded to CBD as positively. Instead, as of mid-2020, the FDA was still expressing its official disapproval of nonpharmaceutical uses of cannabidiol. Simply put, the FDA is not in the business of approving herbal products as medicine. In an updated Consumer Advisory statement that generated alarmist mainstream media headlines about the dangers of CBD, the FDA stated: "CBD has the potential to harm you," noting that it "has seen only limited data about CBD safety and these data point to real risks that need to be considered before taking CBD for any reason."[38]

The administration also dispatched warning letters to 15 CBD companies for "illegally selling products containing cannabidiol (CBD) in ways that violate the Federal Food, Drug, and Cosmetic Act (FD&C Act)" by marketing CBD to treat specific diseases.

> The FDA is not in the business of approving herbal products as medicine.

What is a consumer to believe when on one hand the WHO says CBD has a "good safety profile," while on the other the FDA says the data point to real risks? Let's look more closely at the FDA's concerns.

CBD versus Epidiolex

The FDA's Consumer Advisory outlined a number of safety concerns about CBD products, including "potential liver injury, interactions with other drugs, drowsiness, diarrhea, and changes in mood." One of the biggest problems with this statement is that it is based upon data about Epidiolex, the pharmaceutical CBD product approved for pediatric epilepsy. While it's true that 10 percent of children with epilepsy, when administered Epidiolex in clinical trials, experienced these adverse side effects, it's not clear that they were actually caused by CBD.

For starters, most of the children taking Epidiolex were also on other potent epilepsy drugs. One of these drugs, valproate, is known to cause liver toxicity with long-term use. Also, Epidiolex contains sucralose, the artificial sweetener marketed under the brand name Splenda. Some studies have indicated that sucralose causes liver damage in laboratory animals.

Other side effects of sucralose, which alters the gut microbiome, include diarrhea and gastrointestinal distress. Irritability, agitation, and other mood changes may be the natural response of a critically ill child on multiple medications. Drowsiness can be caused by very large doses of CBD (like the amount used in the Epidiolex trials), but it may also have been caused by the ethanol that Epidiolex contains as a carrier agent. Including sucralose and ethanol in a medicine for sick children is a head-scratcher, but that wasn't an issue for the FDA.

Also, it's important to remember that huge doses of Epidiolex are prescribed to curb seizures; the recommended dose of Epidiolex would be equivalent to a 150-pound adult taking as much as 1,400 mg of CBD daily, which is far more than the vast majority of CBD consumers actually take. That makes a big difference. Drug interactions are much more likely if one consumes large doses of a CBD isolate like Epidiolex. But most people are taking far smaller doses of isolate products and/or are taking even smaller doses of oil extracts that contain a full spectrum of cannabis components, including a tiny amount of THC, in addition to CBD.

CBD and Sperm Production

The FDA statement also said, "Studies in animals have shown that CBD can interfere with the development and function of testes and sperm, decrease testosterone levels and impair sexual behavior in males." Actually "studies" is an exaggeration. The FDA referenced a single study from 1986, which examined whether plant cannabinoids had a negative impact on the fertility of male mice.

Interestingly, this study seemed to exonerate THC: "Males exposed to...THC appeared to have spermatozoa in number comparable to controls." But a large dose of CBD, unlike THC, "reduced the percentage of successful impregnations by cannabinoid-exposed males."[39] This hardly proves that CBD has a negative effect on fertility.

As we have emphasized, extrapolating from animal studies to humans—or choosing not to—is a tricky business, given that mice and people metabolize CBD differently. There is currently insufficient evidence to assert that CBD has a direct (negative or positive) effect on sperm count.

A Few Side Effects

There are very few serious side effects directly linked to CBD (as opposed to Epidiolex, which contains alcohol and an artificial sweetener). To the extent that CBD causes side effects, they are relatively minor, including:

Dry mouth: This is a side effect that is relatively common among cannabis users, and, according to a 2006 study published in *Experimental Biology and Medicine*, is likely due to the saliva-inhibiting effect that cannabinoids have via the CB receptors in our salivary glands.[40] There's an easy fix for this: Be sure to drink plenty of water before and after you consume your CBD oil.

Dehydration: Hemp and cannabis are astringent botanicals. Dehydration could be an issue for any astringent botanical that is consumed on a regular basis. Again, make sure you stay on top of your daily hydration to avoid this issue.

Hypotension: Cannabis is a hypotensive herb; it can lower blood pressure. That's good news if you suffer from high blood pressure, as many people do. But if you have low blood pressure, you might want to monitor your blood pressure when trying CBD products and/or increasing your dose.

CBD and Drug interactions

Drug interactions are a significant consideration in modern medicine. More than half of U.S. adults regularly take prescription meds, and at least 75 percent of Americans take at least one over-the-counter drug. Many people, including most seniors (the fastest growing demographic of cannabis product users), take multiple drugs, and these compounds can interact and affect the metabolism of each other.

Drug interactions can be both useful and dangerous. A drug that interacts with an opiate or a chemotherapy agent could increase the risk of a lethal overdose. But a CBD-rich cannabis product—which has its own painkilling properties while also potentiating the effects of an opiate—could reduce the amount of opiate necessary for pain relief, thereby decreasing the likelihood of an overdose. For purposes of safety, you obviously want to avoid dangerous interactions.

CBD is not intrinsically dangerous; it is only as dangerous as the drug that it interacts with. Dangerous drug interactions are much more likely with high-dose CBD therapy than with other forms of cannabis consumption. Physicians and consumers should be concerned about this, given that the federal regulatory policy prioritizes CBD isolates over plant-derived, multicomponent formulations. Again, dosing definitely matters here, and when you use larger doses (as is often necessary for isolate products), you're more likely to run into problems with interactions.

The way cannabinoids are consumed—whether vaporized, eaten, rubbed on the skin, and so forth—adds another layer to the complexity of drug interactions. The manner in which you consume CBD affects the maximal amount of cannabinoids in the liver and how quickly they get there. Depending on the method you choose, you may want to time your CBD intake so as to not interfere with other medications.

Inhaled cannabinoids via vaping or smoking will go through the lungs (where the drug-metabolizing CYP1 enzyme family is present) into the bloodstream, directly toward the brain and heart. Then they will slowly pass through the liver. Changes in drug metabolism are highly unlikely when CBD is inhaled since the amount of CBD consumed this way is relatively low; but if they occur at all, they would likely begin shortly after inhalation. Several hours after smoking or vaping, the risk of any drug interactions will be much lower.

Ingested cannabinoids are primarily absorbed through the intestines (where the drug-metabolizing enzyme CYP3A is present)

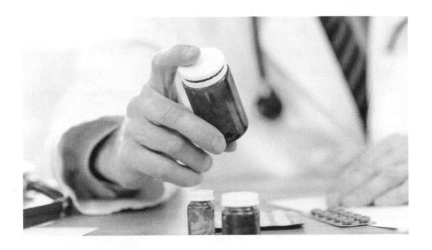

and then are processed by the liver before being distributed through the body. Cannabinoids are more bioavailable, meaning you'll be able to absorb more of the total amount you eat if you take them on a full stomach, but they will absorb more slowly, meaning it will take a longer time for them to get into your system. The time it takes to be processed by the liver and absorbed into the bloodstream usually ranges from 2 to 4 hours. You will have higher peak liver concentrations of cannabinoids if you ingest them rather than inhale them, so ingested cannabinoids will have a greater effect on CYP3A-metabolized drugs (which account for about 30 percent of pharmaceuticals), as they interact with CYP3A in both the intestines and liver.

Oral-mucosal and sublingual CBD administration is a middle ground between inhalation and ingestion. If taken correctly without swallowing, oral-mucosal drugs are absorbed into the bloodstream through membranes in the mouth, along the cheek, and under the tongue. These come in the form of tinctures and under-the-tongue sprays, among other delivery systems. When administered sublingually, cannabinoids aren't immediately processed by the liver—like ingested drugs—but neither do they go directly to the brain and heart—like inhaled drugs. They are just absorbed into the bloodstream.

Sublingual cannabis tinctures take around two hours to reach maximum concentrations in your liver and bloodstream.

Although topical cannabinoids can be absorbed through the skin into joints, they do not get into the bloodstream, so there is no potential for harmful (or helpful) drug interactions. Transdermal administration of cannabinoids, however, is quite different than a regular topical application. A transdermal patch will slowly release cannabinoids into the bloodstream, usually at a constant rate. As with sublingual and inhaled cannabinoids, the liver concentration of cannabinoids administered transdermally should roughly parallel their concentration in the blood.

As a general rule of thumb, if your medications include a grapefruit warning, you should be mindful of possible CBD/drug interactions, since chemicals in grapefruit known as furanocoumarins inhibit CYP34A4 in a similar mechanism as CBD. Those drugs include (but are not limited to) some blood pressure medications, blood thinners, corticosteroids, immunosuppressants, and antidepressants.

Talk to your doctor about how to space out your medication and CBD dosages so they do not interfere with one another. For more information, see Project CBD's "Primer on Cannabinoid-Drug Interactions (https://www.projectcbd.org/how-to/cbd-drug-interactions).

CBD for Special Populations

As CBD increases in popularity, more people from all walks of life are reaching for it for health and wellness purposes. Some have raised concerns about potential risks in special populations like pregnant women, kids, and older adults. Here's what you should know.

CBD in Pregnancy

Although CBD doesn't damage DNA and is neither *mutagenic* (known to harm cells and cause disease like cancer) or *teratogenic* (known to cause birth defects), the FDA has warned women not to use CBD while pregnant or breastfeeding. "What is the effect of CBD on the developing brain?" the FDA asks.

Actually, there is no evidence that CBD harms the brain, developing or otherwise. Federally funded research found that CBD and THC are both neuroprotective antioxidants that promote brain health.

But is CBD a safe choice for pregnant women? When confounding variables like alcohol and tobacco use are accounted for, thus far no reviews have produced evidence that CBD or cannabis alone cause harm to the fetus, as Project CBD documented in a report to California's Office of Environmental Health Hazard Assessment.[41]

Among the key findings:

- There is insufficient evidence to conclude that maternal cannabis use causes long-term adverse developmental outcomes.
- Labeling cannabis, cannabis extracts, cannabis smoke, CBD, or THC as reproductive toxins is not justifiable from high-quality scientific evidence and would misdirect public health and harm-reduction efforts away from known teratogens, like alcohol and tobacco.
- Although cannabinoids are not intrinsically toxic, they may amplify the toxic effects of alcohol, nicotine, and other teratogens. Public health messages should be tailored toward pregnant women using multiple substances.

Moreover, cannabis has been used as a birthing aid to ease pain and facilitate labor contractions in many cultures for centuries. That said, organizations such as the American College of Obstetricians and Gynecologists and the American Academy of Pediatrics maintain a cautious stance on any and all cannabis products, including CBD oil during pregnancy, and recommend that women who are pregnant or contemplating pregnancy should not use cannabis or any of its derivatives.

As is the case with so many issues surrounding CBD and

An Interview with a Cannabis Scientist

Jahan Marcu, PhD

Cannabis is widely recognized as being a safe substance. But it's still important that the cannabis industry has well-thought-out, established regulations and standards for safety for the products that people consume.

Martin A. Lee of Project CBD interviewed Jahan Marcu, PhD, editor in chief of the *American Journal of Endocannabinoid Medicine* and a scientific advisor to Project CBD. This edited conversation addresses what the cannabis industry is doing to ensure safe cannabis-based products like CBD.[42]

Project CBD: *What is a "standard" in the case of cannabis safety protocols?*

Marcu: Similar standards that you'd expect when you buy a salad at a grocery store or you buy a pack of vitamin C—you'd expect a certain level of safety.

Standards usually begin as a best practice. What makes a good manufacturer? A good cultivator? A good dispensary? What makes a good laboratory? A lot of medical cannabis users are looking for something that's going to be consistent.

Project CBD: *How do you establish standards that are going to be applicable nationally when it's only in certain states that cannabis is legal?*

Marcu: American Herbal Products Association (AHPA) and other standards groups have gotten involved because they are not controlled by the DEA. It's not the first time that a substance from a plant has been discovered and made into a legal medicine. You might remember the poppy plant, and opium and morphine. We discovered another endogenous system by investigating that plant.

Project CBD: *Let's talk about testing. Through your work with the Patient Focused Certification (PFC) program of Americans for Safe Access, you've been involved in auditing these labs. What do you see in the labs?*

Marcu: Some of the labs are absolutely ready to be regulated. Some already have inspections from state agencies. Like Washington State; they have some inspectors coming in.

Generally, the labs need to get on board with "best practices." Some labs have done a great job in observing this.

Other labs want to create their own standards. In order for things to be scientifically valid, things to be consistent, laboratories have to get on board with agreeing on some set of standards.

Project CBD: *There's an ISO-certified lab. What does ISO stand for? Is that a kind of a certification that is top of the line?*

Marcu: ISO is an international standard. Having an ISO compliance or being accredited will definitely help you pass a Patient Focused Certification (PFC) audit, because it will make the review of the data methodology much easier. You'll have updated standard operating procedures. But I also look at training records, licensing, zoning, at how you dispose of your waste. We also look at batch tracking and adverse events reporting, making sure that you know who extracted what and what did it go into and where did it go, so that if there's an issue, the product can be tracked or recalled.

The community needs to be its own FDA, in this regard. We have to be vigilant.

cannabis-related products, more research needs to be done. In the meantime, you can make an informed, thoughtful decision based on what we know now, says Stacey Kerr, MD, a teacher, physician, and author based in Northern California. After several years working with the Society of Cannabis Clinicians, and codeveloping the first comprehensive online course in cannabinoid medicine, Kerr became the medical director for Hawaiian Ethos, a vertically integrated cannabis company on the Big Island. Her advice to pregnant women:

- Cannabis can be abused. Don't abuse it.
- Smoke is an irritant to the airways. If you choose to use cannabis, vaporize flowers or use non-smoked products from trusted sources.
- Be clear about why you are using it and re-evaluate those reasons each time.
- Federal law still prohibits cannabis.
- Hospitals, physicians, and social services can have punitive responses to parents who test positive for THC.
- Babies exposed to cannabis during gestation may weigh less than babies not exposed (although for a woman experiencing painful labor, that may not be a detriment).
- Use organic herb and concentrates that are clear of chemicals and pesticides.

CBD and Seniors

Nearly 20 percent of Americans 50 and older said they use CBD products according to a 2019 Gallup Poll.[43] That's not at all surprising when you consider the myriad chronic conditions such as heart disease, dementia, and pain that CBD, if used wisely, is good for. Of course, people in this demographic may also have more confounding factors, such as taking other medications and impaired metabolism and organ function, leading some to wonder if there are specific precautions older adults should take when consuming CBD.

The primary concern would indeed be unwanted drug interactions. Check which of your medications may interact with CBD (see "CBD and Drug Interactions," page 185), and work with your doctor and/or take precautions to avoid potentially harmful interactions.

Polypharmacy is a serious issue for many people, particularly seniors. You may be looking to wean off some of your pharmaceutical or over-the-counter drugs for pain, sleep, or mood disorders like depression. You want to use a more natural product like CBD instead. It's important to not just stop taking any medication and replace it with CBD. That can backfire with a worsening of symptoms. Work with your doctor to taper off one drug as you dial in your dose of CBD to find what works for you.

> Nearly 20 percent of Americans 50 and older said they use CBD products.

The same holds true for CBD-rich cannabis (with more than 0.3 percent THC) obtained via a licensed dispensary, as seniors are currently the fastest-growing demographic of cannabis users worldwide. Israeli researchers addressed questions regarding the safety of cannabis use among seniors in a prospective observational study that involved 184 elderly patients at a geriatric clinic in Israel. Eighty-three percent of the patients were 75 years or older.[44]

Lead researcher Dr. Ilya Reznik discussed their findings at the International Association for Cannabinoid Medicines conference in 2019. The study entailed a comprehensive examination of each participant at the outset of cannabis therapy, plus a follow-up evaluation six months later. None of the participants enrolled in the study had any previous experience with cannabis. Most suffered from chronic pain (77 percent) and other age-related conditions, such as sleep disturbances, cancer-related symptoms, mood disorders, and Parkinson's disease.

The majority of the participants (66 percent) used CBD-rich

cannabis oil sublingually as the sole method of administration, and half of them took three doses daily. For the most part, side effects were relatively mild, affecting one-third of the seniors enrolled in the study; these included dizziness (12 percent), sleepiness (11 percent), and dryness of the mouth.

Most significantly, the six-month follow-up appraisal revealed that one-third of the cannabis patients were able to discontinue opioids, as well as other pharmaceutical painkillers and anti-inflammatory drugs.

Overall, the research and clinical experiences reported at IACM 2019 confirmed the strong safety profile of cannabis-based medication for the senior population, especially when THC levels are balanced by appropriate or equal levels of CBD and the remedies are administered sublingually. Scientists and doctors have also observed promising results with cannabis therapy that may help to improve the quality of life of older adults by mitigating normal as well as disease-based age-related decline. For senior citizens, that means improvement in cognition and mobility, increased body weight, decreased constipation, and better overall functioning.[45]

CBD and Kids

Currently, the only FDA-approved CBD product is being used to treat children (specifically for severe cases of epilepsy). So, it's natural that parents would be curious about the benefits of CBD for their kids, especially for children with difficult to manage conditions like autism, as well as mood disorders like anxiety.

It's a tricky subject. Pioneer cannabis clinicians like pediatrician Bonni Goldstein, MD, author of *Cannabis Is Medicine*, caution against marijuana use in teens. "In most healthy children, their endocannabinoid system is functioning, and actually adding cannabis to that endocannabinoid system may interfere with developing brains," she told Project CBD.[46] "So, I don't encourage teenagers—and I'm the mom of a teenage boy—to use cannabis." If one is going to use cannabis recreationally, it's better to wait until they are older and their brain is fully developed, she advises.

But it's another story, according to Goldstein, when you're dealing with unhealthy kids with diseases that indicate that their endocannabinoid system is dysfunctional. "Healthy kids are not coming to a doctor for help with cannabis," she explains. "It's the children that are sick. And, in my practice, I'm seeing the sickest of the sick. I'm seeing children who have intractable epilepsy, which means they're not responding to any treatment that's available. And there are some aggressive treatments—brain surgery, special diets that are very difficult to keep, lots of different medications that have toxic side effects. I'm also seeing children with autism. And we know, really there is no medicine for autism. There's therapy, which can be very helpful, but there's only two approved medications, and both of them are antipsychotics, not great for children (many bad side effects). As well as children with cancer. And also I'm seeing some children with severe psychiatric disease where current conventional medication hasn't helped," she says.

The issue then for certain children is that the endocannabinoid system, which helps with homeostasis and keeps the brain in balance,

CBD Behind the Wheel

The FDA issued a bulletin on December 18, 2019, "Taking Cannabidiol (CBD) Products and Driving Can Be Dangerous," which warned people not to drive a motor vehicle under the influence of CBD. The basis for this bulletin was research conducted on children who were heavily medicated with benzodiazepines and became drowsy after receiving a large dose of CBD. And very high doses (exceeding 1,000 mg) of CBD may have a sedating effect. But CBD by itself in the quantities that most people take has never been shown to be intoxicating or impair coordination or perception and has never been linked to hazardous driving.

can actually be the core of the problem for kids with certain illnesses, as Goldstein explains: "These are children who sometimes are not finding the answers. Years go by, and when you lose years of a child's life, you're losing development, quality of life—the burden of illness is tremendous not only for the child but for the whole family."

In those cases, experienced practitioners like Goldstein will work with kids. "We're giving measured doses of CBD oil to children, again starting based on weight, low dose, titrating up, looking for that child's sweet spot. And sometimes less is better than more. Sometimes we hit a point, we say, 'Oh no, we did much better at a lower dose,' and we back down."

Goldstein has seen no downsides to this type of treatment, even when the doses are above the sweet spot. "Because the tolerance is so good, there are no negative side effects really. I've even had the experience of three particular patients over the last few years where a parent that measured wrong on the syringe and overdosed their children. The child had a very nice nap! Slept all night, and really there was no downside," she says.

If you want to use CBD to manage a child's health issue, it's best to work with your pediatrician so they know what the child is taking, especially if the child is on other medications.

CHAPTER

11

Your CBD
Action Plan

ETERMINING THE OPTIMAL amount of any given CBD product to take may require a lot of trial and error. But knowing the general bioavailability of each type and how quickly each method works can help you devise a CBD plan of action following these steps:

Step 1: Choose the form(s) of CBD you want to try.

Step 2: Research specific CBD products.

Step 3: Consult with your doctor.

Step 4: Experiment with dosing and timing.

Step 5: Track your results.

Step 1: Choose the Form(s) of CBD You Want to Try

The form you decide to use depends on the reasons you want to use CBD. For instance, if you want to use CBD for anxiety, you could use a few drops of a daily tincture to lower your overall symptoms, and use a faster-acting method like a vape pen or nasal mist for acute anxiety attacks when you need quick relief. For arthritis pain, you may find that you can lower your inflammation and keep flare-ups in check with regular use of edibles or other slower-acting, longer-lasting forms, and use additional topical CBD products directly over painful joints as needed.

In a nutshell, CBD products that are processed through the digestive system, such as gummies and capsules, take longer (up to 2 hours) to take effect but also are long lasting (up to 12 hours). Those that go straight into your bloodstream, such as under-the-tongue tinctures, vapes, and topicals are fast acting but also don't last quite as long.

Also consider the type of product you're most comfortable taking. If you hate the taste of tinctures, you'll be less likely to want to use them consistently. If you're on the go a lot, it might be most convenient for you to have a pack of gummies in your purse or pocket. Think about the form that fits best into your lifestyle.

See Chapter 7 for details on each form of CBD.

Step 2: Research Specific CBD Products

Because the CBD marketplace is as regulated as the Wild West, it's important to do your research to find a quality product. The manufacturer should openly provide detailed information about the products they sell, including:

Type of product: Full-spectrum, isolate, etc.

What is in the bottle: Cannabinoids, carrier oils, terpenes, and any other ingredients.

Third-party lab testing & quality assurance: The manufacturer should be able to provide Certificate of Analysis from a third-party testing facility.

If the manufacturer is not completely transparent about these important details, shop elsewhere. Also, review the information in Chapter 8 about where to shop, what to buy, and how to read labels.

"I Tried It"

Anna Symonds, 38,
Portland, Oregon

At age 38, Anna Symonds is in her 18th year of playing in the USA Rugby Women's Premier League (WPL). "Despite being ancient by the competitive standards of my sport," she says, "my physical conditioning and overall health are at the best of my adult life. I'm still competing at the top level of the U.S. domestic women's competition—and I'm convinced that the healing properties of CBD and cannabis, along with a nourishing diet and regular therapeutic movement, are crucial to my success and longevity as an athlete."

Before games, Symonds takes full-spectrum CBD-rich supplements for "precovery," to optimize her physical, mental, and emotional condition so she can perform at a peak level.

Immediately after a game, she uses CBD to combat inflammation, along with THC as needed for acute pain. (She lives in Oregon, where cannabis is legal.) She may smoke a preroll or use a vape cartridge for this recovery and, if possible, will take a CBD-infused Epsom salt bath so that she can feel muscle relief penetrating from outside as well as inside.

When she had sports hernia surgery several years ago, she says, "I used only full-spectrum cannabis and CBD products in my post-op recovery, and it went as well as I could have hoped—my healing was quick, the pain was manageable, and I was much more functional than the previous time I had surgery."[47]

It's also helpful to know where and how the CBD plants were grown and how the CBD oil was extracted, but this information may not be readily available. Look for American organically (and preferably regeneratively) grown hemp or cannabis. European hemp regulations are geared toward fiber and seed oil plants, not high-resin, CBD-rich cultivars. And poorly regulated Chinese hemp is not subject to strict environmental standards.

Pesticide-laden hemp grown in polluted soil is not a good source of CBD, as heavy metals and other toxins are concentrated in the oil extracted from plants grown in suboptimal conditions. Industrial-scale CBD oil extraction also increases the risk of unhealthy solvent residues in your CBD product. Toxic solvent residues are less likely in oil extracted using ethanol or supercritical CO_2 technology.

If your doctor is open to and knowledgeable about CBD and cannabis therapeutics, he or she should be your first stop when considering what kind of CBD product is right for you. Trusted, experienced friends and/or family members also can help point you in the right direction.

Otherwise, if you're not sure where to start, search online for "CBD Oil Near Me." (This should point you to nearby licensed dispensaries (if cannabis is legal in your state), as well as stores that only sell hemp-derived CBD products. That will give you a chance to find an establishment where you can take your time, browse, and ask questions about the products that interest you. Project CBD also maintains a list of licensed cannabis dispensaries and hemp CBD stores at https://www.projectcbd.org/find-cbd/dispensaries.

Step 3: Consult with Your Doctor

Millions of people use CBD as part of their daily wellness regimen. If you are interested in using CBD to treat a specific medical condition, consult your doctor (or a doctor who has knowledge of and experience with CBD).

Because high doses of CBD can interact with and maybe dangerously amplify (or block) the effects of a number of commonly used medications, an experienced medical professional can help you dial in your CBD use in a way that will minimize problematic drug interactions. For example, you could take your medications in the morning and your CBD in the evening. As a rule of thumb, that includes any medications with a "grapefruit warning," since chemicals in grapefruit known as furanocoumarins inhibit CYP34A4 in a similar mechanism as CBD. Those drugs include (but are not limited to) blood pressure medications, blood thinners, corticosteroids, immunosuppressants, and antidepressants. For more information on this subject, see Project CBD's "Primer on Cannabinoid-Drug Interactions." (https://www.projectcbd.org/how-to/cbd-drug-interactions).

CBD for Exercise and Sports

Whether you run 5-Ks, go to the local CrossFit gym, or play tennis on the weekends, you know that lingering muscle inflammation from exercise can hinder performance.

That's why CBD has become a star player in the sports and exercise world. Professional and amateur athletes alike are crediting CBD lotions, tinctures, and fortified supplements with helping them recover faster. Their muscles feel fresher faster, they heal injuries more quickly, and they play pain-free. CBD manufacturers are also increasingly partnering with pro athletes and event promoters like Spartan, the obstacle course racing company.

That's not surprising when you consider some of the consequences of using traditional pain relievers. Chronic use of over-the-counter pain relievers like NSAIDs are hard on the gut, tax the liver and kidneys, and may actually slow the recovery process, where your muscles mend themselves to come back stronger.

There is currently no research on how CBD can hasten recovery and/or improve exercise performance. But given what we do know, there's reason to believe that it can help. CBD acts as an anti-inflammatory, can help us feel less pain, and can improve sleep quality, all of which go a long way in helping you recover and feel less sore following hard workouts.

Some athletes also believe that CBD can help them get in "the zone" or achieve a "flow state" more easily, where exercise feels effortless and they're completely tuned into the task at hand. CBD interacts with key neurotransmitters in the brain that trigger the runner's high sensation and the calming effects people can get from exercise. In a similar way, a CBD supplement could make your next yoga session or Spin class even more enjoyable.

Bottom line: If you keep a medicine cabinet full of "vitamin I" (aka ibuprofen) handy for everyday aches and pains related to exercise, you may want to put down the ibuprofen and acetaminophen and try CBD. It's easier on your GI system and may have bonus benefits of speeding recovery and making exercise feel easier.

According to Bonni Goldstein, MD, a Los Angeles–based physician, author of *Cannabis Is Medicine*, and the medical director of Canna-Centers, "Patients suffering with inflammation have many choices when it comes to cannabis medicine. Along with the ability to choose 'nonsmokable' delivery methods, such as tinctures, edibles, topical balms, and vaporizers, patients now have many choices of which combination of cannabinoids to use.

"One can take cannabis medicine that is THC-rich, CBD-rich, combination CBD+THC, THCA, CBDA, and/or CBG. Some cannabis medicine suppliers are combining raw and heated cannabinoids in tinctures to increase the anti-inflammatory benefits. Many patients are benefitting from drinking the juice of raw cannabis plants. In my medical practice, I have seen thousands of patients eliminate or reduce the need for NSAIDs, reducing their risks of side effects and possibly even death, with the use of cannabis," she says.[48]

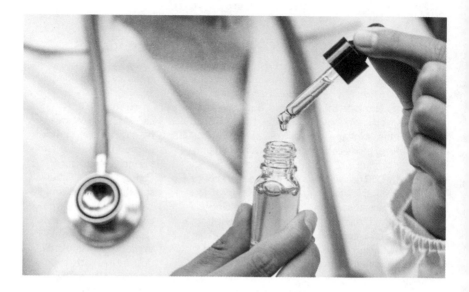

The following are some tips for consulting with a medical professional regarding CBD:

- **Explain why you're interested.** Be clear and upfront about what you're looking to use CBD for. For instance, you could say, "My arthritis seems to be getting worse, and I have read that CBD oil can help," or "I've been having some problems with anxiety lately, and my research shows that CBD has helped people with anxiety."
- **Bring along some evidence.** Bring along this book! Or you can bring other well-researched documents you found showing evidence that CBD can provide the benefits you're looking for.
- **Ask for help integrating CBD into your treatment plan.** Your doctor should be monitoring your progress on your current medications and/or health plan. Ask them to help you work CBD into that plan.
- **Seek a second opinion, if necessary.** You and your doctor should be on the same team striving for your best health. If your doctor is not willing to discuss or learn about CBD, find

one who is. The Society of Cannabis Clinicians has an online resource that can help you find one near you: https://www.cannabisclinicians.org/find-a-cannabis-doctor/.

Step 4: Experiment with Dosing and Timing

Remember the golden rule with cannabis therapeutics: Start low and go slow. Once you find the right dose, you can also manipulate and adapt the timing of your doses to meet your needs. Lower doses can be energizing, while larger doses can make you sleepy, so if you take larger daily doses, you can divide them accordingly to get the effects you desire without side effects that you don't. Review the guidelines in the Chapter 9 guide you in this trial-and-error process.

Step 5: Track Your Results

Because CBD works differently for different people, it's a good idea to track your results to help you figure out the best methods, timing, and dosing for you. Use the tracking sheet on the following page to help you. Photocopy it as many times as needed.

My CBD Tracker

Date: _____

Symptoms: _____

CBD product taken: _____

___ Full-spectrum   ___ Intranasal
___ Broad-spectrum Isolate   ___ Transdermal
___ Distillate   ___ Suppository
___ Oral   ___ High potency
___ Sublingual   ___ Medium potency
___ Topical   ___ Low potency
___ Inhaled

THC%: _____   CBD %: _____

Dose taken: _____

Time taken: _____

Time to feel effects: _____

Effects: _____

_____

Time effects wore off: _____

Other medications or supplements taken: _____

_____

Food/drink: _____

Notes: _____

_____

_____

12

CBD Recipes

W HILE THERE IS a vast marketplace of CBD concentrates and edibles in state-licensed dispensaries and online storefronts, there are several reasons to consider making your own infused concentrates in the form of tinctures and butters to add to food and drink.

Ensure quality: While there are many legitimate companies producing high-quality, third-party lab-tested products, there are also many hyping questionable goods—and the lack of FDA regulation of the CBD marketplace makes it hard to know the difference. Making your own concentrates and edibles ensures a clean, high-quality final product.

Save money: Making your own cannabis products is inexpensive—often significantly cheaper than similar products found in dispensaries, and they'll be fresher and taste great, too.

Reap benefits of the whole plant: Cooking with the whole cannabis plant, regardless of whether the strain is high in CBD or THC, can better retain more of the valuable terpenes—the compounds in cannabis that provide the aroma, flavor, and nuance inherent in the plant that will ultimately influence the body's response.

Hide the flavor: Pot brownies might make you think of the Summer of Love, but those flower children knew what they were doing. Some people just aren't crazy about the taste of whole-plant cannabis con-

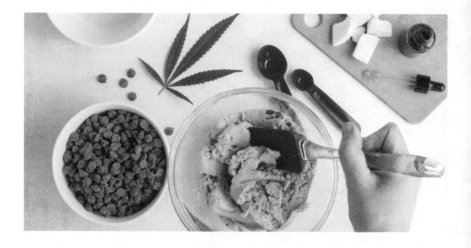

centrates, and chocolate is a great foil for covering its herbal flavors, as are aromatic herbs, spices, and other potent flavorings.

Go raw: Adding raw cannabis flowers to smoothies, pesto, and other recipes allows you to incorporate the many benefits of raw cannabis into your food. Move over, kale!

Make it personal: The cannabis plant, with its vast offering of possibilities of health benefits, naturally invites your participation. Making your own medicine and treats can be a truly satisfying experience. You'll get to know each product's unique qualities and effects and develop a deeper understanding and appreciation for all CBD and its entourage has to offer.

In this chapter, we've included several recipes for CBD-rich medicinal tinctures, CBD-rich topicals, and CBD-infused edibles. Each of these recipes, developed by Melinda Misuraca for Project CBD, can be easily adapted to utilize whatever cannabis products are legal and/or available to you—whether whole dried flowers, full-spectrum CBD-rich oil extracts or broad-spectrum oil without THC, or medicinal concentrates that include a healthy amount of both CBD and THC in states where this is legal. Another option: Use a CBD isolate as an all-purpose add-in ingredient to one of your own favorite recipes.

Decarboxylation

You will see that some of the recipes below call for dried CBD-rich cannabis flowers (hemp or marijuana) either raw or decarboxylated. Decarboxylation entails heating cannabis to convert the cannabinoids from their raw "acid" form (e.g., CBDA, THCA) that's present in the plant into a neutral form (CBD, THC). To date, most of the studies into the therapeutic effects of cannabinoids have used decarbed cannabis. Though research into the benefits of raw, unheated cannabinoids is still new, there may be some conditions for which raw CBD-rich cannabis is warranted. More research is needed.

To decarb, preheat the oven to 220°F. Grind dried cannabis flowers to a fine consistency in a spice or coffee grinder, and spread on a parchment-lined baking sheet. Bake for 45 minutes. Let cool.

Equipment

Making your own CBD edibles and remedies doesn't require a lot of fancy equipment, but it will certainly help to gather what you need ahead of time.

To make the tinctures in this chapter, you will need:
• kitchen scale
• spice or coffee grinder
• 3 wide-mouth canning jars with tight-fitting lids
• fine mesh strainer, cheesecloth, or coffee filter
• funnel
• 1- or 2-ounce amber or other dark color glass bottles

To make the topicals in this chapter, you will need:
• kitchen scale
• spice/coffee grinder
• measuring cups and spoons
• spatula
• double boiler and/or slow cooker

- fine mesh strainer or cheesecloth
- one medium glass jar
- several small glass jars for finished oil and topicals (preferably amber or other dark color)

To make the edibles in this chapter, you will need:
- slow cooker
- cheesecloth
- sieve or colander
- large heat-proof bowl
- heat-proof rubber spatula
- large-size silicone gummy molds (enough to make 24 gummies)
- small saucepan
- measuring cups and spoons
- whisk
- cookie sheet
- airtight container or zip-top bags
- spice grinder or mortar and pestle
- quart-sized canning jar
- wooden spoon
- small metal funnel
- glass dropper bottles
- labels

Ingredients

Some of the ingredients in the following recipes are common kitchen staples, but others may not be as familiar. In general, you can find herbs and essential oils at most community markets, health food stores, and online shops. Two good online sources are www.mountainroseherbs.com and www.bulkapothecary.com.

10 Ways You Can Use Cannabis in the Kitchen

1. Make a batch of CBD-rich cannabutter to use in baked treats!

2. Add cannabis-infused olive oil to salad dressing, drizzle over veggies, toss into a pasta dish, or stir into soups, sautés, and spaghetti sauce.

3. Grind dry, decarboxylated cannabis flowers in a spice grinder, and mix in your favorite spices to make a special spice blend. Try sprinkling it on popcorn!

4. Make a delicious CBD chai tea blend by mixing 3 cups water with 1 g CBD-rich ground or finely chopped dried raw cannabis flowers; 1 tsp butter or coconut oil; 1 small cinnamon stick; a few each of cloves, peppercorns and cardamom pods; and a few slices of ginger. Bring to a boil, then turn down and simmer until reduced to 2 cups, about 10 minutes. Strain and add milk and honey or sugar to taste.

5. Make CBD ice cream! Use your favorite recipe, and infuse the cream beforehand by heating approximately 1 g whole dried raw flowers (chopped or ground) per cup of heavy cream. Infuse in a heavy-bottom saucepan at low heat for 10 minutes. Cool and continue the recipe.

6. Make pesto, replacing some of the basil with fresh hemp or other cannabis shade leaves.

7. Add cannabis shade leaves to your favorite smoothie recipe instead of kale.

8. Make your own cannabis-infused gummies or jellies.

9. Make cannabis-infused bitters by steeping ¼ oz CBD-rich cannabis flowers (along with ¼ cup dried hibiscus flowers; 2 tsp each dried orange peel, dried lemon peel, and dried ginger root; 1 tsp crushed cardamom seeds; and ¼ cup dried sour cherries, all finely chopped) in 2 cups of vodka, rum, or another grain alcohol for 2 weeks, then strain.

Heat ¾ cup of sugar on medium-high on the stove top until caramelized, add it to the mixture, and stir until dissolved.

10. Make CBD-infused chocolate mousse, custards, puddings, and other cream-based desserts by infusing the cream with CBD-rich cannabis before continuing the recipe.

Note:

If you can't or don't want to make your own concentrates, you can still buy a high-quality CBD oil or extract and add it to your favorite recipe.

The main thing to consider when adding cannabis to foods and drinks is potency and dosage. Recipes using flowers from hemp or a high-CBD strain with a negligible amount of THC (0.3 percent or lower) or raw cannabis flowers or shade leaves means that the chance of getting high is pretty slim.

Please label ALL cannabis edibles, and keep away from children.

CBD-Rich Tincture for Inflammation and Pain

Studies show that CBD's anti-inflammatory and analgesic properties can effectively ease pain conditions that are often treated with OTC drugs. When combined with potent herbs—like ginger,[49] turmeric,[50] boswellia,[51] and white willow bark[52]—that provide similar properties, CBD can knock pain down to size.

MAKES:
approximately four 2-oz or eight 1-oz dropper bottles of tincture

INGREDIENTS:

1-oz bottle of full- or broad-spectrum CBD oil containing 1,500 mg CBD OR ¼-½ oz CBD-rich cannabis flowers (raw or decarboxylated)

¼ oz dried ginger

¼ oz turmeric powder

¼ oz dried boswellia

¼ oz dried white willow bark

½ tsp ground black pepper

8–12 oz high-proof alcohol, like Everclear or pure grain alcohol OR 8–12 oz vegetable glycerine

DIRECTIONS:

To extract your herbs (including CBD-rich cannabis flowers, if using), choose one of the following three extraction methods:

1. **Slow alcohol tincture method:** This is the best choice, as alcohol is the most effective solvent, and using the slow, no-heat method is safe and makes the most potent extract.

2. **Fast alcohol tincture method:** Uses excellent solvent properties but uses heat for a super-fast extraction when you just don't have a month to wait around. Must be careful to monitor the process and keep heat stable.

3. **Glycerine tincture method:** Good choice for those who want an alcohol-free extract relatively quickly (in 24 hours).

For all three methods, follow these first two steps:

1. Grind herbs. Place all plant matter, including cannabis flowers (if using), in wide-mouth pint or quart canning jar.

2. Add alcohol or glycerine as necessary to completely cover herbs as they absorb liquid. Seal jar tightly with lid.

3. Follow next step according to extraction method you chose:

   a. **Slow alcohol tincture method:** Place jar in dark, dry place; and shake every 2 to 3 days, adding more alcohol if needed to cover herbs. After steeping for 4 weeks, move on to Step 4.

   b. **Fast alcohol tincture method:** Heat deep pot filled with water to 170°F. Place cannabis/alcohol jar in pot, and allow to heat for 30 minutes to an hour, keeping temperature stable. Remove from pot and let cool for at least an hour. Move on to Step 4.

   c. **Glycerine tincture method:** Place washcloth or folded towel in bottom of slow cooker, and fill halfway with warm water. Place sealed jar of glycerine and herbs in slow cooker, place lid on top if it still fits (otherwise drape kitchen towel over it), and set to warm for 24 hours. Shake jar occasionally to disperse ingredients. Use pot holder to take jar from slow cooker, and let jar cool for at least an hour. Move on to Step 4.

4. Place fine sieve or several layers of cheesecloth or coffee filter secured with rubber band over clean bowl, and strain out plant material. With clean hands, twist cheesecloth, and squeeze remaining liquid from herbs. If there's more sediment left than you'd like, cover and allow to settle overnight and then strain again through coffee filter.

5. Add cannabis extract, if using, and mix well. Use funnel to decant into small 1-oz or 2-oz dark glass bottles. Label, date, and store in cool, dark place. Alcohol-based tinctures can last for years. Vegetable glycerine tinctures last about a year and are best kept in refrigerator when not in use.

HOW TO USE:
Adult dosages are typically 10–50 drops in water or tea three times a day as needed. Start with the lower dosage, see how you feel, and adjust accordingly.

Calculating a Dose
That Contains an Extract

If you made your tincture with a CBD oil extract, you can calculate a specific standard dose. First, measure the amount of finished tincture. Let's say you ended up with 8 oz, or 237 mL (rounded off). Then divide the amount of cannabinoids you added. In this case, divide 1,500 mg CBD by 237; you end up with 6.3 mg/mL. Generally, there are 20 drops in a mL, but you should test it with your dropper. A moderate dose of CBD is between 5 and 15 mg, so 6.3 mg is a good amount. As always, start low and go slow.

CBD-Rich Tincture for Sleep

CBD's antianxiety and stress-relieving benefits blend well with herbs known for their calming, sleep-inducing properties, such as chamomile, valerian, and California poppy (a specific poppy species known for its anxiolytic effects). If you live in a state where it is legal, you may want to try using some THC-rich flowers or oil along with your CBD-rich material for this recipe. A 1:1 ratio of CBD to THC can be very effective for sleep.

MAKES:
approximately four 2-oz or eight 1-oz dropper bottles of tincture

INGREDIENTS:

1-oz bottle of full- or broad-spectrum CBD oil containing 1,500 mg CBD OR ¼-½ oz CBD-rich cannabis flowers (raw or decarboxylated)

⅛ oz dried ginger

⅛ oz dried passionflower

⅛ oz dried chamomile

⅛ oz dried valerian

⅛ oz dried hops

⅛ oz dried California poppy

⅛ oz dried lemon balm

8–12 oz high-proof alcohol, like Everclear or pure grain alcohol OR 8–12 oz vegetable glycerine

DIRECTIONS:
To extract your herbs (including CBD-rich cannabis flowers, if using), choose one of the following three extraction methods:

1. **Slow alcohol tincture method:** This is the best choice, as alcohol is the most effective solvent, and using the slow, no-heat method is safe and makes the most potent extract.

2. **Fast alcohol tincture method:** Uses excellent solvent properties but uses heat for a super-fast extraction when you just don't have a month to wait around. Must be careful to monitor the process and keep heat stable.

3. **Glycerine tincture method:** Good choice for those who want an alcohol-free extract relatively quickly (in 24 hours).

For all three methods, follow these first two steps:

1. Grind herbs. Place all plant matter, including cannabis flowers (if using), in wide-mouth pint or quart canning jar.

2. Add alcohol or glycerine as necessary to completely cover herbs as they absorb liquid. Seal jar tightly with lid.

3. Follow next step according to extraction method you chose:

   a. **Slow alcohol tincture method:** Place jar in dark, dry place; and shake every 2 to 3 days, adding more alcohol if needed to cover herbs. After steeping for 4 weeks, move on to Step 4.

   b. **Fast alcohol tincture method:** Heat deep pot filled with water to 170°F. Place cannabis/alcohol jar in pot, and allow to heat for 30 minutes to an hour, keeping temperature stable. Remove from pot and let cool for at least an hour. Move on to Step 4.

   c. **Glycerine tincture method:** Place washcloth or folded towel in bottom of slow cooker, and fill halfway with warm water. Place sealed jar of glycerine and herbs in slow cooker, place lid on top if it still fits (otherwise drape kitchen towel over it), and set to warm for 24 hours. Shake jar occasionally to disperse ingredients. Use pot holder to take jar from slow cooker, and let jar cool for at least an hour. Move on to Step 4.

4. Place fine sieve or several layers of cheesecloth or coffee filter secured with rubber band over clean bowl, and strain out plant material. With clean hands, twist cheesecloth, and squeeze remaining liquid from herbs. If there's more sediment left than you'd like, cover and allow to settle overnight and then strain again through coffee filter.

5. Add cannabis extract, if using, and mix well. Use funnel to decant into small 1-oz or 2-oz dark glass bottles. Label, date, and store in cool, dark place. Alcohol-based tinctures can last for years. Vegetable glycerine tinctures last about a year and are best kept in refrigerator when not in use.

HOW TO USE:
A typical adult dose is 10–50 drops. Take the dose about an hour before bed. Start with a low dosage of around 10 drops; wait half an hour to see how you feel. Adjust accordingly.

Note: This recipe is best for someone who has used CBD before and is familiar with how it interacts with their body's unique biology. Though it's rare, CBD can be stimulating for some people. If you are one of those people, you might try using the CBD-rich stress tincture throughout the day; studies have shown that CBD taken during the day can help with nighttime insomnia.[53]

CBD-Rich Tincture for Stress

The traditional Ayurvedic herbs ashwagandha and holy basil have been shown to calm the body by regulating the stress hormone cortisol, while lemon balm improves mood and cognitive performance, and bacopa helps protect the brain against the ravages of stress. Add the proven stress-busting properties of CBD, and you have a powerful brain elixir for these modern times.

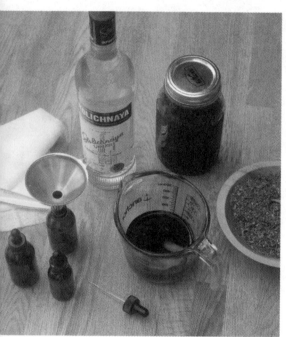

MAKES:
approximately four 2-oz or eight 1-oz dropper bottles of tincture

INGREDIENTS:
1-oz bottle of full- or broad-spectrum CBD oil containing 1,500 mg CBD OR ¼-½ oz CBD-rich cannabis flowers (raw or decarboxylated)

¼ oz dried ashwagandha

¼ oz dried holy basil

¼ oz dried lemon balm

¼ oz dried bacopa

8–12 oz high-proof alcohol, like Everclear or pure grain alcohol OR 8–12 oz vegetable glycerin

DIRECTIONS:
To extract your herbs (including CBD-rich cannabis flowers, if using), choose one of the following three extraction methods:

1. **Slow alcohol tincture method:** This is the best choice, as alcohol is the most effective solvent, and using the slow, no-heat method is safe and makes the most potent extract.

2. Fast alcohol tincture method: Uses excellent solvent properties but uses heat for a super-fast extraction when you just don't have a month to wait around. Must be careful to monitor the process and keep heat stable.

3. Glycerine tincture method: Good choice for those who want an alcohol-free extract relatively quickly (in 24 hours).

For all three methods, follow these first two steps:

1. Grind herbs. Place all plant matter, including cannabis flowers (if using), in wide-mouth pint or quart canning jar.

2. Add alcohol or glycerine as necessary to completely cover herbs as they absorb liquid. Seal jar tightly with lid.

3. Follow next step according to extraction method you chose:

    a. Slow alcohol tincture method: Place jar in dark, dry place; and shake every 2 to 3 days, adding more alcohol if needed to cover herbs. After steeping for 4 weeks, move on to Step 4.

    b. Fast alcohol tincture method: Heat deep pot filled with water to 170°F. Place cannabis/alcohol jar in pot, and allow to heat for 30 minutes to an hour, keeping temperature stable. Remove from pot and let cool for at least an hour. Move on to Step 4.

    c. Glycerine tincture method: Place washcloth or folded towel in bottom of slow cooker, and fill halfway with warm water. Place sealed jar of glycerine and herbs in slow cooker, place lid on top if it still fits (otherwise drape kitchen towel over it), and set to warm for 24 hours. Shake occasionally to disperse ingredients. Use pot holder to take jar from slow cooker, and let jar cool for at least an hour. Move on to Step 4.

4. Place fine sieve or several layers of cheesecloth or coffee filter secured with rubber band over clean bowl, and strain out plant material. With clean hands, twist cheesecloth, and squeeze remaining liquid from herbs. If there's more sediment left than you'd like, cover and allow to settle overnight and then strain again through coffee filter.

5. Add cannabis extract, if using, and mix well. Use funnel to decant into small 1-oz or 2-oz dark glass bottles. Label, date, and store in cool, dark place. Alcohol-based tinctures can last for years. Vegetable glycerine tinctures last about a year and are best kept in refrigerator when not in use.

HOW TO USE:
Adult dosages are typically 10–50 drops in water or tea, three times a day as needed. Start with the lower dosage, see how you feel, and adjust accordingly.

CBD Topical Base Oil

This CBD base oil recipe makes enough for the creams and salves in this chapter with plenty left over. You can also apply the oil as is directly on the skin for many dermatological issues. To extend freshness, keep unused oil sealed tightly in the fridge for up to a year. The calendula, chamomile, and Arnica montana flowers are anti-inflammatory (the first two also aid in wound healing), while St. John's wort flowers are antimicrobial.

MAKES:
about 2 cups

INGREDIENTS:
1 cup virgin coconut oil

1 cup cold-pressed almond oil

¼ oz dried calendula flowers

¼ oz dried chamomile flowers

OPTIONAL:
¼ oz dried *Arnica montana flowers*

¼ oz St. John's wort flowers

CHOOSE EITHER:
1-oz bottle of full- or broad-spectrum CBD oil containing 1,500 mg CBD OR ¼-½ oz CBD-rich cannabis flowers (raw or decarboxylated)

DIRECTIONS:
1. Grind herbs, then place all plant matter (including cannabis flower) with coconut and almond oils in slow cooker or yogurt maker. Let infuse for 12 hours or overnight at lowest heat setting. Alternatively, place all plant matter and coconut and almond oil in double boiler filled with 2–3 in. water, and let simmer for 3–4 hours, adding more water as needed.

2. With fine-mesh strainer or several layers of cheesecloth rubber-banded over clean bowl, strain out all plant material, squeezing out remaining oil with clean hands if using cheesecloth.

3. If using CBD oil as additive or base ingredient, add now and mix well.

4. Store your cannabis topical base oil in clean jar, labeled, dated, and placed in cool, dark place. Keep out of reach of children.

CBD-Rich Anti-Itch Cream

This soothing cream relies on the anti-inflammatory properties of CBD to help calm the skin, combined with other ingredients known for their antibacterial, antiseptic, pain-relieving, and healing properties, such as witch hazel, apple cider vinegar, peppermint essential oil, and tea tree oil. Lavender oil is anti-inflammatory as well as antiseptic.

MAKES:
about 1½ cups

INGREDIENTS:

½ cup CBD topical base oil

2 Tbsp shea butter

2–3 Tbsp beeswax pellets or finely chopped beeswax

3 Tbsp baking soda

½ cup bentonite clay, pink kaolin clay, or a half-and-half mix

2 tsp witch hazel

2 tsp apple cider vinegar

20 drops peppermint essential oil

10 drops tea tree oil

10 drops lavender oil

DIRECTIONS:

1. Using double boiler or heat-safe bowl that can sit in pot with about 2 inches of water, heat infused topical base oil and shea butter over low to medium heat. Add beeswax and stir until dissolved.

2. Remove from heat and add baking soda, bentonite clay, witch hazel, and apple cider vinegar to mixture. Add peppermint, tea tree, and lavender oils. Blend well.

3. Place spoonful into freezer for 2 minutes, then check consistency. If too thin, melt some more beeswax pellets over low heat in separate pan and mix in.

4. Pour or spoon cream into jar with tight-fitting lid, label, date, and store in cool, dark place. As it continues to cool, cream should solidify into spreadable consistency.

HOW TO USE:
Apply to inflamed, itchy skin as needed. For external use only. Not intended for mucous membranes or genital areas. Discontinue if skin becomes more irritated.

CBD and Mānuka Honey Antibiotic Salve

Both CBD and mānuka honey are potent allies against bacterial infections, including methicillin-resistant Staphylococcus aureus (MRSA) infections. Along with witch hazel and essential oils known for their antiseptic and antimicrobial properties, they combine to make a healing, bug-fighting salve, a powerful ally against topical infections of all kinds.

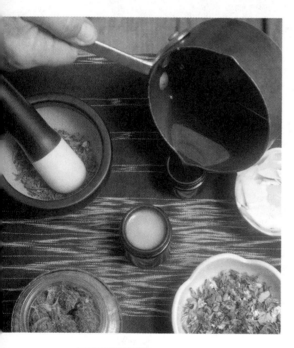

MAKES:
about ¾ cup

INGREDIENTS:

½ cup CBD topical base oil

1 Tbsp shea butter

2–3 Tbsp beeswax pellets or finely chopped beeswax

1 Tbsp raw New Zealand mānuka honey

1 tsp witch hazel

6 drops tea tree oil

6 drops lavender oil

6 drops thyme oil

6 drops oregano oil

DIRECTIONS:

1. Heat CBD topical base oil in double boiler until just warm.

2. Add shea butter and beeswax and stir until dissolved.

3. Remove from heat and let cool until lukewarm.

4. Add mānuka honey and essential oils and stir until thoroughly mixed.

5. Pour into small glass jars, label, date, and store in cool, dark place.

HOW TO USE:
Due to the honey, this salve is a bit sticky. Apply a thin layer of salve over a clean, superficial wound or any area where you might have contracted a bacterial skin infection. This is not intended to be used on deep or puncture wounds.

Mānuka Honey

Other types of honey also have antibacterial properties, but mānuka is the only honey that has been shown to be powerful enough to kill staph. Bees make it with nectar collected from the tea tree plant, which is indigenous to New Zealand. Mānuka honey can be purchased online. One should look for mānuka honey with a certified potency rating of at least UMF 15 or higher, which indicates its antibacterial strength.

CBD-Rich Inflammation and Pain Relief Balm for Muscles and Joints

This balm is designed to penetrate below the skin and into deeper tissues, with transdermal help from natural permeability enhancers such as menthol, eucalyptus, and camphor—aromatic ingredients that also have analgesic properties.

MAKES:
about ¾ cup

INGREDIENTS:
½ cup CBD topical base oil

1 Tbsp shea butter

2–3 Tbsp beeswax pellets, or clean beeswax, chopped fine

1 Tbsp menthol crystals

6 drops eucalyptus essential oil

6 drops camphor oil

DIRECTIONS:
1. Heat CBD topical oil in double boiler until just warm. Add shea butter, beeswax, and menthol crystals and stir until dissolved.

2. Remove from heat and let cool until lukewarm.

3. Add eucalyptus and camphor oils and stir until thoroughly mixed.

4. Pour into small glass jars, label, date, and store in cool, dark place.

HOW TO USE:
Apply liberally to affected areas, and rub in until completely absorbed. Use as needed. Discontinue if irritation or allergic reaction occurs.

CBD-Rich Nourishing Facial Oil

Given CBD's antioxidant, antibacterial, and anti-inflammatory properties, it is a perfect skin care ingredient. For this recipe, you'll want to use a CBD-rich extract that is mixed with a medium-chain triglyceride (MCT) oil (typically derived from coconut oil); it should be labeled as such. An alcohol-based tincture would be too drying for your skin.

MAKES:
approximately 2 ½-3 oz (depending on the diluted strength of the CBD extract)

INGREDIENTS:
½ oz (1 Tbsp) jojoba oil

½ oz (1 Tbsp) sweet almond oil

½ oz (1 Tbsp) apricot kernel oil

¼ oz (½ Tbsp) rosehip oil

¼ oz (½ Tbsp) argan oil

½ -1 oz CBD-rich full-spectrum extract in an MCT oil base, equivalent to approximately 600 mg CBD

OPTIONAL:
6–8 drops each of one to three essential oils for fragrance and skin-nourishing properties. Some suggestions:

jasmine (antioxidant, wound-healing, antimicrobial)

tangerine, orange, lemon, neroli (anticancer; increases skin absorption)

lavender (anti-inflammatory)

rose (antioxidant)

clary sage (antioxidant, antimicrobial)

frankincense (anti-inflammatory, wound-healing)

sandalwood (anti-inflammatory, antimicrobial)

chamomile (soothes irritations)

DIRECTIONS:
Mix all ingredients together in ceramic, glass, or stainless steel bowl. Store in dark glass dropper bottle in cool, dark place.

HOW TO USE:
A little goes a long way. Too much and you can gum up your skin barrier. This oil is best used first thing in the morning or before bed, 4–6 drops for face and neck and a little more for décolletage (chest) area. Dot your fingers with oil, rub together lightly, then gently pat on freshly cleansed face and neck, lifting often to distribute to other areas. Wait a few minutes for your skin to absorb the oil before applying other skin products or getting dressed. One recipe should last you 2 to 3 months with regular use.

Cannabutter

Infusing butter (or coconut oil for a vegan product) with CBD oil or CBD-rich flowers will result in a final product rich with plant terpenes. This gives cannabutter a herbaceous flavor that is pleasant to some, though not so much to others. But fear not! There are many ways to downplay and even hide the flavor if you so desire.

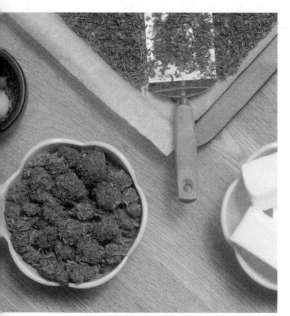

MAKES:
approximately 2 lb butter

INGREDIENTS:
1-oz bottle of full- or broad-spectrum CBD oil containing 1,500 mg CBD OR ½-1 oz CBD-rich cannabis flowers (raw or decarboxylated)

2 lb unsalted butter or unrefined coconut oil

1 qt hot tap water

DIRECTIONS:
1. Coarsely grind dried cannabis in hand grinder, mortar and pestle, or coffee grinder (if using latter, make sure to grind it coarsely)

2. Place all ingredients in slow cooker set on low. Once it heats, allow to cook for 8–24 hours. Add extra water if level falls too low.

3. Line colander or sieve with cheesecloth and place over heatproof bowl. Pour cannabutter through and let drain for 10 minutes. Gather cheesecloth, and with spatula, wooden spoon, and/or clean hands, press out remaining butter.

4. Cover bowl and chill in fridge until butter (or coconut oil) has solidified, about 3–4 hours or overnight.

5. Remove cannabutter from bowl, discard water, and pat butter or solid oil dry with paper towels. Don't worry about small bits of cannabis left behind in butter—they'll mix in.

6. Store cannabutter in airtight container or zip-top bags in fridge for up to 2 weeks or in freezer for up to 6 months. Use in your favorite baked treats!

Bite-Size CBD-Rich Fudgy Brownies

These yummy morsels are a delicious way to incorporate CBD into your diet. Made with terpene-rich cannabutter, the chocolate is an excellent foil for mellowing the herbaceous flavor of cannabis. If stored in the freezer, you can take one out as needed—they taste just as good frozen, too. If you use THC-rich cannabutter, use half cannabutter and half regular unsalted butter for a less potent brownie.

MAKES:
36 bite-size servings

INGREDIENTS:

10 Tbsp (140 g) CBD-rich cannabutter

1¼ cups (250 g) granulated sugar

¾ cup plus 2 Tbsp (65 g, may vary by brands) unsweetened cocoa powder (natural or Dutch-processed)

¼ tsp kosher salt

½ tsp pure vanilla extract

2 large eggs, cold

½ cup (65 g) all-purpose flour

⅔ cup (75 g) walnut or pecan pieces, toasted (optional)

DIRECTIONS:

1. Position rack in lower third of oven and preheat oven to 325°F. Line bottom and sides of 8-inch square baking pan with parchment paper or foil for easy removal.

2. Combine butter, sugar, cocoa, and salt in medium-size heatproof bowl.

3. Set bowl over saucepan of simmering water. Stir occasionally with heatproof spatula until butter is melted and mixture is smooth and hot to touch.

4. Remove bowl from heat and cool until mixture is just warm, with gritty texture.

5. Stir in vanilla. Add eggs, one at a time, stirring well after each one. Add flour and beat vigorously for 40 strokes, until mixture is smooth and glossy. Stir in nuts, if using. Spread evenly in lined pan.

6. Bake until toothpick inserted into brownies emerges slightly moist with batter, 25-30 minutes. Let cool completely on rack.

7. Remove brownies by lifting up two sides of parchment or foil and place on cookie sheet. Freeze for half an hour or until firm.

8. With sharp knife, cut into 36 squares. Wrap each square in waxed paper or foil, and store in an airtight container or zip-top bag in refrigerator or freezer. Keeps for 1–2 weeks in fridge or 6 months in freezer.

CBD-Infused Hibiscus-Berry Gummies

These fat-free, super-fruity gummies are an easy, delicious way to dose CBD and can even be made with stevia or monk fruit extract for a sugar-free version. Berries and hibiscus are rich in healthful polyphenols and combine to create a lovely deep red color. Hibiscus flowers are easy to find in Mexican markets or health food stores. You can either buy dried raspberry or strawberry powder or make your own by grinding freeze-dried berries in a spice grinder. You can also substitute agar for the gelatin, but follow package directions.

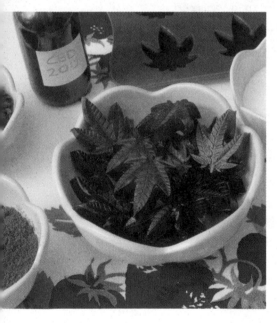

MAKES:
about 24 large gummies

INGREDIENTS:
¾ cup water

¼ cup dried hibiscus flowers
(or 6 hibiscus tea bags)

3 Tbsp dried raspberry or strawberry powder

1½ Tbsp sugar OR 2 Tbsp honey
OR 2 Tbsp agave OR ½–1 tsp stevia or
monk fruit extract (to taste)

1 Tbsp fresh lemon or lime juice
OR ¼– ½ tsp vitamin C powder for ex-
tra-sour gummies

4 Tbsp unflavored gelatin

CBD-rich tincture, purchased or homemade
(see page 210, 212, or 214), measured to
accurately dose 24 servings (see Note on the
next page)

DIRECTIONS:
1. Boil water and pour ¾ cup over hibiscus flowers or tea bags in heatproof cup or bowl. Let steep for 5 minutes. Strain out flowers and measure out ¾ cup tea.
2. Combine all ingredients except gelatin and CBD extract in small saucepan over medium-low heat. Stir with whisk.

3. Cook until hot but not boiling. Gently sprinkle gelatin over top of mixture a little at a time, whisking constantly until completely mixed in.

4. Continue stirring, cooking over medium-low heat until gelatin has completely melted and fruit mixture is smooth and glassy.

5. Remove from heat. Add CBD-infused tincture and mix thoroughly.

6. Place gummy mold on a cookie sheet and carefully fill with mixture using small measuring cup, spoon, or dropper.

7. Chill in fridge until firm, approximately 2 hours, using toothpick to pierce any air bubbles that appear.

8. Carefully release gummies from mold. For denser, chewier gummies, let air-dry for a day on wire rack in dry room. Store finished gummies in airtight container in fridge. Keeps up to 2 weeks.

Note: Any alcohol- or glycerine-based CBD-rich tincture can be used for this recipe. Figure out your individual dose (5–10 drops, for example) and multiply by 24. Half a dropper typically contains 20 drops. Add this amount to the mixture after gelatin is dissolved.

CHAPTER

13

CBD for Pets

W HEN A DOG or a cat gets sick and conventional options don't work, people seek alternatives. CBD is one that a lot of people are exploring. One 2019 survey reported that 39 percent of dog owners and 34 percent of cat owners approved of the idea of CBD for pets. Twenty-nine percent of the survey takers were interested in purchasing CBD pet supplements, and 11 percent of dog owners and 8 percent of cat owners had already given CBD- or hemp-infused treats to their pets.[54]

But questions abound. In an industry so poorly regulated when it comes to products designed for human consumption, how do we know what we're buying for our pets? Is it safe? And is it worth it?

We'll answer these questions and give some basic guidelines to pet owners in this chapter, which is adapted with permission from articles written for Project CBD by Gary Richter, DVM, an integrative medicine veterinarian based in Oakland, California, and founder of Holistic Veterinary Care and co-founder of the Veterinary Cannabis Society.

What Science Says So Far

One thing we do know is that all vertebrates (that is, any animal that has a backbone)—including amphibians, reptiles, birds, fish, and mammals—have an endocannabinoid system.

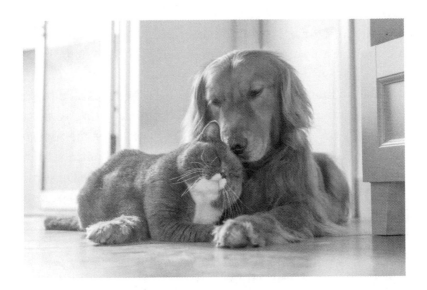

From what we know so far, the endocannabinoid system in a dog or a cat is similar to that of a human. One striking difference is that there appears to be a greater concentration of cannabinoid receptors in the dog's brain than there are in most other animals. This is significant because it makes dogs more susceptible to THC overdose. THC can be dangerous to dogs, potentially causing some neurologic impairment in the short term. Otherwise, when cannabis medicine is used effectively, their endocannabinoid system will act in the same way it would for a human.

Currently, pain relief is the most well documented of all the uses of cannabis-based treatments in veterinary medicine. A growing number of veterinarians and pet owners have seen the positive effects of medical cannabis for the treatment of arthritis and other forms of pain in animals. Research trials confirm those experiences, showing profound pain-relieving effects from cannabis-based products like CBD for a variety of medical conditions.

In one 2018 study published in *Frontiers in Veterinary Science*, Cornell University researchers showed that dogs with osteoarthritis that were given 2 mg/kg of CBD twice a day enjoyed a significant reduction in pain and increase in activity with no negative side effects.[55]

As it does in humans, CBD may also help reduce the frequency and severity of seizures in dogs with epilepsy, according to a study published in the June 2019 issue of the *Journal of the American Veterinary Medical Association*.[56] The study of 16 pet dogs led by neurologist Stephanie McGrath, DVM, of Colorado State University's James L. Voss Veterinary Teaching Hospital found that 89 percent of dogs that received CBD significantly reduced the frequency of seizures.

"It's really exciting that perhaps we can start looking at CBD in the future as an alternative to existing anticonvulsive drugs," McGrath said in a statement on the study.

Scientific evidence for CBD benefits for cats is harder to come by.[57] So far, research indicates that it is generally safe, but cats appear to need different dosing and product strategies than dogs. In a small study on the effects of a single dose of CBD-rich hemp on cats and dogs published in the journal *Animals*, cats ultimately ended up with about one-fifth as much CBD in their systems following dosing than dogs. Felines also were more resistant to taking CBD, showing "excessive licking and head-shaking during oil administration," according to the study (in which case, it might help to add it to their food and see if they accept it better that way).

Both pet owners and researchers are interested in how CBD may help alleviate anxiety in pets, but those studies are still forthcoming.[58] Anecdotally, vets have found animals can benefit from medical cannabis for many of the same reasons it helps people, including anxiety, pain, and seizures, as well as gastrointestinal disorders, inflammation, and cancer.

Unfortunately, it can be challenging to find trusted, educated individuals who can provide professional guidance on cannabinoid therapies for pets. In a recent survey of more than 2,000 veterinarians, less than half of them were comfortable talking to their clients about CBD for pets. Among this group, vets were most comfortable recommending CBD for pain management, anxiety, and seizures in dogs. And among those who had experience treating pets with CBD, the vast majority (~80 percent) did not feel that state veterinary organizations provide enough guidance on how to abide by state or federal laws. A similar proportion believed that from a moral and medical perspective, CBD should be allowed for pets.[59]

"I Tried It"

Cash, 10,
Kingston, New Hampshire

Cash is a German Shorthaired Pointer. He's a classic hunting dog. Gunshots in the outskirts of his home in Kingston, New Hampshire? No sweat. (Or shakes!) Fireworks, on the other hand? Before his owners found CBD, a few festive explosions in the neighborhood would send poor Cash into a tizzy of whining, panting, shaking, and quaking.

"It started about four years ago," his owner, Michael Dobrowolski, says. "People in this town love their fireworks, and Cash developed a lot of anxiety around them."

Dobrowolski and his wife tried everything to no avail. "We tried thunder vests, wrapping him in a blanket, turning up the TV and radio; nothing seemed to work."

Then they came across some information on CBD for pets and figured it was worth a shot. "It took a little trial and error before we found a brand that worked. But eventually we found one that is a soft, chewable treat that really takes the edge off and dramatically reduces his anxiety," Dobrowolski says.

Each treat contains 3 mg of CBD, and Dobrowolski gives him just a couple according to the dosing instructions on the label (1 chewable for every 30 pounds). In 30 to 45 minutes, the dog calms down.

"He's still himself. It's not like he's drugged or subdued. He's alert and on point, but he's very chill and much more relaxed. It's pretty cool," Dobrowolski says.

Obviously, the chews work best if you can give them in advance of the booms, bangs, and fireworks, Dobrowolski says. "But even if I give them to him when the noise begins, they still help. You just have to be patient while you wait for them to kick in."

CBD FOR PETS

To help pet owners become better informed about the use of cannabis-based products like CBD for their four-legged companions, Project CBD compiled the following guidelines with the assistance of Dr. Richter.

How to Choose the Right Form for Your Pet

Medical cannabis-based products like CBD for pets usually come as a liquid or as treats. Liquids are preferable because the dosing can be accurately controlled and because CBD may be better absorbed through the tissues of the mouth rather than through the digestive tract.

Vaporized or smoked cannabis should never be used with pets. This can damage their lungs and can lead to accidental overdose.

Similarly, edibles for humans should not be given to your pet, because they are impossible to dose accurately and they may contain ingredients (such as raisins and chocolate) that are toxic to animals. Plant materials should be kept away from pets.

How to Choose the Right Medicine

When considering cannabis-based treatment for your pet, it is important to understand how the various components of a cannabis preparation may affect your pet. Some important factors to keep in mind are:

Choose CBD products for pets. CBD products for pets are similar to those made for humans, but they are not the same. For one, they may be flavored differently to appeal to your pet, such as using cod liver oil for CBD oil for cats because they'll like it better. You can find CBD products specially designed for cats, dogs, horses, birds, and other pets. They are easy to find online, but it's especially important to do your due diligence and choose a manufacturer that can provide a certificate of analysis (COA) and provide details about the products' quality just as you would for yourself.

The entourage effect: Just as with humans, a whole-plant product for your pet is best because of the synergistic benefit of the major and minor cannabinoids, terpenes, and flavonoids.

The right ratio: Use the appropriate ratio of THC and CBD as well as dosage. Ratios of THC to CBD frequently range from as high as 40:1, to even ratios (1:1), to 1:40. In general, the more severe the pain, the more THC will help.

When using cannabis as medicine for pets, the first thing to remember is that any significant side effects are unacceptable. Getting your dog or cat stoned is never okay, even with medical cannabis. The goal with cannabis therapy in pets is to relieve the symptom being treated with no other side effects. Their normal patterns of behavior should be unaltered after receiving the therapy.

Quality control: Do your due diligence. Call the company and ask where the product is coming from and how it's being produced. There is no government oversight to make sure that these companies are selling authentic and safe products. Ideally, you would look for a product that is organic and produced locally. You want to know how much CBD and THC are present.

Legal status: Cannabis is federally illegal across the board. Regulations regarding what veterinarians are able to discuss with pet owners regarding cannabis varies from state to state. As of September 2020, however, veterinarians cannot provide a medical marijuana recommendation.

Other medications: Consider other medications being given concurrently with respect to possible drug interactions. These are similar to the medications that can have interactions in people, including anti-inflammatories and antidepressants.[60] And always consult with your veterinarian before beginning any new medication or supplement for your pet. As you would with your own doctor, explain clearly why you're interested in exploring CBD for your pet,

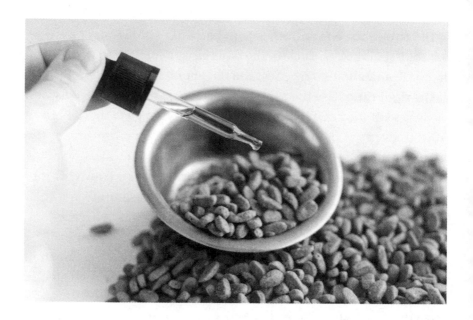

and bring along any research you may have done on the subject. (See page 202 for more tips on consulting with your medical professional.) If you feel that your vet is not being open-minded, you may need to seek a second opinion.

Dosage Guide for Pets in Pain

As with people, it's best to begin at the low end. Start with 0.5 mg of CBD per 10 pounds of body weight twice daily. If needed, slowly increase the dose every 4 to 7 days. Frequently, doses nearer the lower end of the range are effective but higher doses may be beneficial in certain circumstances. you've achieved the desired effect for whatever is being treated, then you're probably done.

If CBD alone isn't effective and you live in a state where cannabis is legal, formulations containing THC may be helpful. Consult with your veterinarian prior to using any product containing THC.

Medical cannabis can be of great benefit to animals in pain.

Ultimately, however, safe and effective use of cannabis requires an understanding of the milligram amounts of THC and CBD (or other cannabinoids), the ratio of cannabinoids, and availability of a medicine in a concentration appropriate for dosing a pet.

Nothing is more important than the safety of your pet, so don't make guesses or assume anything about the content or dosing of cannabis medicines.

Glossary

Biphasic effect: Many compounds, including CBD, produce a biphasic effect, meaning that low and high doses can produce opposite effects.

Broad-spectrum: Broad-spectrum CBD-rich oil is the essential oil from cannabis minus the tetrahydrocannabinol (THC). It is designed to provide the entourage effect from combining CBD with other cannabinoids and terpenes without the potential high or risk of failing a drug test.

Cannabidiol: The scientific name of CBD, a naturally occurring compound extracted from cannabis plants, which has a broad range of actions including reducing anxiety, inflammation, and stress, among other myriad health benefits.

Cannabigerol: The scientific name of CBG, another cannabinoid found in the cannabis plant that has medicinal value as an analgesic, anti-inflammatory, antidepressant, bone stimulant, and cancer-fighting molecule.

Cannabis: A family of flowering plants including hemp plants that contain little to no THC (but generally contain CBD) and drug plants that contain higher amounts of THC, as well as CBD.

CBDA: The acidic, raw form of CBD that exists in the CBD-rich cannabis plant before it has been dried and heated. It may be more effective against some conditions than CBD or THC.

CBD distillate: A cocktail of different isolates that may contain as much as 80 percent CBD along with small amounts of other cannabinoids and terpenes.

CBD isolate: An isolate means the product contains just CBD and nothing else from the plant. There is no entourage effect with isolates.

COA: Abbreviation for certificate of analysis; a third-party certification that shows how a cannabis product performed on screenings for CBD, THC, and any contaminants.

CYP enzyme: The family of enzymes that break down drugs and other substances in your liver, which is responsible for CBD metabolism.

Endocannabinoid: A naturally occurring molecule made by the body that attaches to cannabinoid receptors and activates them like a key turning a lock. The two best studied endocannabinoids are 2-Arachidonoylglycerol (2AG) and anandamide.

Endocannabinoid system: ECS for short, the endocannabinoid system plays a major role in brain function, immune activity, and maintenance of equilibrium in our organ systems. Dysfunction of the ECS underlies many major diseases.

Entourage effect: Also known as the ensemble effect, this describes the way myriad compounds magnify the benefits of each other. For instance, CBD and THC interact with all the other cannabinoids and terpenes in the cannabis plant so that the medicinal impact of the whole plant is greater than the sum of its parts.

Epidiolex: A CBD-based pharmaceutical drug that has been approved by the FDA for the treatment of certain types of seizure disorders.

GLOSSARY

Extraction: The way in which CBD and other beneficial components are removed from the plant in a highly concentrated form. There are various extraction techniques for CBD, including CO2, hydrocarbon, and ethanol.

Full-spectrum CBD: Sometimes called "whole-plant," full-spectrum means that the product contains the full essential oil in ratios and concentrations that are extracted from the plant, including CBD, THC, terpenes, and other cannabinoids.

Hemp: A cannabis plant with 0.3 percent THC or less.

Hemp seed: The seeds of the hemp plant. Protein-rich hemp seed oil contains omega-3 fatty acids and other healthful compounds, but it contains no CBD, no THC, and no plant cannabinoids to speak of.

Marijuana: The flower of a cannabis plant that contains more than 0.3 percent THC.

Metabolic enzyme: Proteins that accelerate chemical reactions. They are involved in both creating endocannabinoids when needed and breaking them down and destroying them once the endocannabinoids have served their purpose.

Nanotechnology: A process that allows CBD manufacturers to create water-soluble (as opposed to the usual fat-soluble) versions of CBD for inclusion in beverages.

Pharmacopoeia: The branch of medical science that studies drugs and medicinal preparations of many cultures throughout history. The United States Pharmacopoeia is a scientific, nonprofit organization that sets standards for the identity, strength, quality, and purity of medicines, dietary supplements, and food ingredients.

Receptors: Miniature portals that sit on the surface of cells throughout our brain, central nervous system, and other organs that pick up important signals in the body. There are two main types of cannabinoid receptors: CB_1 and CB_2.

Resin: A sticky tar-like residue on plants. In cannabis plants, the resin is found mainly on the plant's flower buds and to a lesser extent on the leaves.

Sativex: A pharmaceutical mucosal spray with nearly equal amounts of CBD and THC.

Sublingual: Designed to be placed under your tongue. Sublingual CBD is one of the quickest and most effective ways to get CBD into your bloodstream.

Terpenes: Aromatic molecules that evaporate easily and create a strong fragrance. Terpenes often have therapeutic benefits and can help cannabinoids like CBD and THC cross the blood–brain barrier and get into your system more easily.

Tetrahydrocannabinol: The scientific name for THC; the compound that causes the high that cannabis is famous for, which works in concert with CBD and also has significant health and wellness benefits.

Tincture: A concentrated herbal extract. CBD is commonly taken in tincture form.

Transport molecule: Known as fatty acid binding proteins, these act like shuttles for endocannabinoids, ferrying them to where they need to go in your body.

Trichomes: Tiny, mushroom-shaped "cannabinoid factories" that cover cannabis flowers. This is where most of the resin and CBD, THC, and other cannabinoids are contained.

Resources

Books & Special Reports

Michael Backes, *Cannabis Pharmacy* (Black Dog & Leventhal, 2017).

Mary Biles, *The CBD Book: The Essential Guide to CBD Oil* (Harper UK, 2020).

Adrian Devitt-Lee, Project CBD's Primer on Cannabinoid-Drug Interactions https://www.projectcbd.org/sites/projectcbd/files/downloads/cannabinoid-drug-inter-actions_2018-10-11.pdf

Bonni Goldstein, MD, Cannabis Is Medicine: *How Medical Cannabis and CBD Are Healing Everything from Anxiety to Chronic Pain* (Little Brown, 2020).

Martin A. Lee, *Smoke Signals: A Social History of Marijuana—Medical, Recreational and Scientific* (Scribner, 2013).

Leonard Leinow and Juliana Birnbaum, *CBD: A Patient's Guide* (North Atlantic, 2017).

Dustin Sulak, DO, *Handbook of Cannabis Clinicians: Principles and Practice* (Norton, 2021)

Linda Parker, *Cannabinoids and the Brain* (MIT Press, 2017).

Cheryl Pellerin, *Healing with Cannabis: The Evolution of the Endocannabinoid System and How Cannabinoids Help Relieve PTSD, Pain, MS, Anxiety, and More* (Skyhorse, 2020).

Jenny Sansouci, *The Rebel's Apothecary: A Practical Guide to the Healing Magic of Cannabis, CBD, and Mushrooms* (TarcherPerigee, 2020).

Jonathan Treasure, *The Thinking Patient's Guide to Cannabis and Cancer* (OncoHerb Press, 2016).

Nishi Whitely, *Chronic Relief: A Guide to Cannabis for the Terminally and Chronically Ill (Alivio LLC, 2016).*

Websites and Organizations

Project CBD (projectcbd.org)
A California-based nonprofit dedicated to promoting and publicizing research into the medical uses of cannabidiol (CBD) and other components of the cannabis plant.

Healer (Healer.com)
An online resource for medical cannabis users, providing cannabis information, education, and online training programs.

Society for Cannabis Clinicians (cannabisclinicians.org)
A nonprofit educational and scientific society of physicians and health care professionals dedicated to the education and research support of cannabis for medical use.

International Cannabinoid Research Society (ICRS) (icrs.co)
Provides an open forum for researchers to meet and discuss their research.

International Association for Cannabinoid Medicine (IACM) (www.cannabis-med.org)
A resource for clinical studies and information regarding the medicinal effects, uses, possible side effects, and the laws and politics of cannabis medicine.

RESOURCES

PubMed (National Library of Medicine) (pubmed.ncbi.nlm.nih.gov)
The website of the National Library of Medicine, which comprises more than 30 million citations for biomedical literature from MEDLINE, life science journals, and online books.

Mary Biles (marybiles.com)
Mary Biles is a medical cannabis writer and educator. Her website includes brand recommendations and medical cannabis news.

American Botanical Council (herbalgram.org)
Also known as the Herbal Medicine Institute, the ABC is an independent, nonprofit research and education organization dedicated to providing accurate and reliable information on the use of herbs and medicinal plants.

Wholistic Research & Education Foundation (wholistic.org)
Dedicated to educating the public and health care practitioners with research-driven data and to helping drive evidence-based drug policy.

Realm of Caring (realmofcaring.org)
A site dedicated to providing research, education, and building community in the realm of cannabis use. Provides access to research, opportunity to enroll in studies, and other educational resources for people and their pets.

American Cannabis Nurses Association (cannabisnurses.org)
Dedicated to advancing excellence in cannabis nursing practice through advocacy, collaboration, education, research, and policy development. Provides education and research resources for people interested in medical cannabis.

NORML (norml.org/)
NORML's mission is to move public opinion sufficiently to legalize the responsible use of marijuana by adults and to serve as an advocate for consumers to assure they have access to high-quality marijuana that is safe, convenient, and affordable. You can find the most up-to-date status of cannabis laws in the United States here.

Americans for Safe Access (ASA) (safeaccessnow.org)
A site dedicated to advancing legal medical marijuana therapeutics and research that includes guides to talking to your doctor, using medical cannabis, and more.

Bulk Apothecary (bulkapothecary.com)
An outlet for bulk herbs, essential oils, waxes, and butters, and other ingredients and equipment for making your own CBD products.

Mountain Rose Herbs (mountainroseherbs.com)
A good source for bulk herbs, essential oils, teas, beeswax, carrier oils, and other ingredients and equipment for making your own CBD products.

Notes

Introduction

1 "2018 Farm Bill Provides a Path Forward for Industrial Hemp," Farm Bureau, Market Intel, February 28, 2019.

2 "US CBD Market to Grow 700% Through 2019," Brightfield Group, July 9, 2019.

3 Marcel O. Bonn-Miller, Mallory J. E. Loflin, Brian F. Thomas, et al., "Labeling Accuracy of Cannabidiol Extracts Sold Online," Journal of the American Medical Association, 318: 17 (2017): 1708-1709.

Part I

1 Sarah Rense, "Here Are All the States That Have Legalized Weed in the U.S.," Esquire (February 7, 2020).

2 Stacey Kerr, " Managing Nausea with Cannabis," Project CBD, February 26, 2018.

3 Cannabis Conversations, "New Developments in Cannabis Medicine with Bonni Goldstein, MD," Project CBD, (March 9, 2020).

4 Kyoung Sang Cho, Young-ran Lim, Kyungho Lee, Jaeseok Lee, Jang Ho Lee, and Im-Soon Lee, "Terpenes from Forests and Human Health," Toxicological Research 33, no. 2 (April 2017): 97–106.

5 Peir Hossein Koulivand, Maryam Khaleghi Ghadiri, and Ali Gorji, "Lavender and the Nervous System," Evidence-Based Complementary and Alternative Medicine (March 14, 2013).

6 Ethan B. Russo, "Taming THC: Potential Cannabis Synergy and Phytocannabinoid-Terpenoid Entourage Effects," British Journal of Pharmacology 163, no. 7 (August 2011): 1344–64.

7 Katrina Weston Green, "The United Chemicals of Cannabis: Beneficial Effects of Cannabis Phytochemicals on the Brain and Cognition," Recent Advances in Canabinoid Research, Willard J. Costain and Robert B. Laprairie, IntechOpen.

8 "Terpenes and the 'Entourage Effect,' " Project CBD.

9 Mary Barna Bridgeman and Daniel T. Abazia, "Medicinal Cannabis: History, Pharmacology, and Implications for the Acute Care Setting," P&T 42, no. 3 (March 2017): 180–88.

10 Jeffrey Gitto, "Potential Legal Pathways for the Sale of Non-psychotropic Cannabanoids," Special Advisory Committee on Cannabis, Silver Springs, MD, May 31, 2019.

11 "Antique Cannabis Book."

12 Martin A. Lee, "Cannabis Oil vs. Hemp Oil," Project CBD.

13 "2018 Farm Bill Provides a Path Forward for Industrial Hemp," Farm Bureau, Market Intel, February 28, 2019.

14 Ernest Small and Arthur Cronquist, "A Practical and Natural Taxonomy for Cannabis," TAXON 25, no. 4 (August 1976): 405–35.

15 Roger G. Pertwee, "Cannabinoid Pharmacology: The First 66 Years," British Journal of Pharmacology 147, suppl. 1 (January 2006): S163–S171.

16 Pál Pacher and George Kunos, "Modulating the Endocannabinoid System in Human Health and Disease: Successes and Failures," FEBS Journal 280, no. 9 (May 2013): 1918–43.

17 V. DiMarzo, D. Melck, T. Bisogno, and L. DePetrocellis, "Endocannabinoids: Endogenous Cannabinoid Receptor Ligands with Neuromodulatory Action," Trends in Neuroscience 22, no. 2 (February 1999): 80.

18 Adrienne Dellwo, "What Is the Endocannabinoid System," verywellhealth (February 10, 2020).

19 D. Fraga, C.I.S. Zinoni, G.A. Rae, C.A. Parada, and G.E.P. Souza, "Endogenous Cannabinoids Induce Fever Through the Activation of CB_1 Receptors," British Journal of Pharmacology 157, no. 8 (August 2009): 1494–1501.

20 Harding, Anne, "I Tried CBD Cream for My Pain: Here's How It Worked," The Healthy (updated August 20, 2020).

21 Hui-Chen Lu and Ken Mackie, "An Introduction to the Endogenous Cannibinoid System," Biological Psychiatry 79, no. 7 (April 1, 2016): 516–25.

22 Fan Hong, Shijia Pan, Yuan Guo, Pengfei Xu, and Yonggong Zhai, "PPARs as Nuclear Receptors for Nutrient and Energy Metabolism," Molecules 24, no. 14 (July 2019): 2545.

23 Joseph Maroon and Jeff Bost, "Review of the Neurological Benefits of Phytocannabinoids," Surgical Neurology International 9 (April 26, 2018): 91.

24 "How CBD Works," Project CBD.

25 Diana McKeon Charkalis, "How CBD Helped One Woman with Anxiety and Sleep Problems," The Healthy, updated August 20, 2020.

26 Wallace, Alicia, "Patent No. 6,630,507: Why the U.S. Government Holds a Patent on Cannabis Plant Compounds," The Denver Post, updated October 2, 2016.

27 Prakash Nagarkatti et al., "Cannabinoids as Novel Anti-Inflammatory Drugs," Future Medicinal Chemistry 1, no. 7 (October 2009): 1333–49.

28 Megan Scudellari, "Your Body Is Teeming with Weed Receptors," The Scientist (July 16, 2017).

29 Jamie Esk, "What Is Oxidative Stress?" Medical News Today (April 3, 2019).

30 James M. Nichols and Barbara L.F. Kaplan, "Immune Responses Regulated by Cannabidiol," Cannabis and Cannabinoid Research 5, no. 1 (2020).

31 Annamaria Vezzani, Jacqueline French, Tamas Bartfai, and Tallie Z. Baram, "The Role of Inflammation in Epilepsy," Nature Reviews. Neurology. 7, no. 1 (January 2011): 31–40.

32 Ryusuke Yoshida et al., "Endocannabinoids Selectively Enhance Sweet Taste," Proceedings of the National Academy of Sciences of the United States of America 107, no. 2 (January 12, 2010): 935–39.

33 James M. Nichols and Barbara L.F. Kaplan, "Immune Responses Regulated by Cannabidiol," Cannabis and Cannabinoid Research 5, no. 1 (2020).

34 Ana Juknat et al., "Cannabidiol Affects the Expression of Genes Involved in Zinc Homeostasis in BV-2 Microglial Cells," Neurochemistry International 61, no. 6 (November 2012): 923–30.

35 Patryk Remiszewski et al., "Chronic Cannabidiol Administration Fails to Diminish Blood Pressure in Rats with Primary and Secondary Hypertension Despite Its Effects on Cardiac and Plasma Endocannabinoid System, Oxidative Stress and Lipid Metabolism," International Journal of Molecular Science 21, no. 4 (February 14, 2020): 1295.

36 Office of the Surgeon General, "Bone Health and Osteoporosis: A Report of the Surgeon General," Rockville (MD): Office of the Surgeon General (US); 2004. 2, The Basics of Bone in Health and Disease.

37 G. Hu, G. Ren, and Y. Shi, "The Putative Cannabinoid Receptor GPR55 Promotes Cancer Cell Proliferation," Oncogene 30 (2011): 139–41.

38 "The Endocannabinoid System & the Biology of Wellness," Project CBD (May 1, 2019).

39 Ethan B. Russo, "Clinical Endocannabinoid Deficiency (CECD): Can This Concept Explain Therapeutic Benefits of Cannabis in Migraine, Fibromyalgia, Irritable Bowel Syndrome and Other Treatment-Resistant Conditions?" Neuroendocrinology Letters 25, nos. 1–2 (February-April 2004): 31–39.

40 Dan Witters and Jim Harter, "Worry and Stress Fuel Record Drop in U.S. Life Satisfaction," Gallup (May 8, 2020).

41 Chokshi, Niraj, "Americans Are Among the Most Stressed People in the World, Poll Finds," The New York Times (April 25, 2019).

42 "Runner's High: Is It Really All Endorphins?" GU.

43 "The Endocannabinoid System & the Biology of Wellness," Project CBD (May 1, 2019).

44 David A. Reichlen, et al., "Wired to Run: Exercise-Induced Endocannabinoid Signaling in Humans and Cursorial Mammals with Implications for the 'Runner's High,'" Journal of Experimental Biology 215 (2012): 1331–36.

45 Mary Biles, "Cannabis, CBD & Anxiety: Could Cannabidiol Help Us Cope During Stressful Times?" Project CBD (May 6, 2020).

46 Donovan A. Argueta, Pedro A. Perez, Alexandros Makriyannis, Nicholas V. DiPatrizio, "Cannabinoid CB1 Receptors Inhibit Gut-Brain Satiation Signaling in Diet-Induced Obesity," Frontiers in Physiology, 2019.

47 Keith A. Sharkey and John W. Wiley, "The Role of the Endocannabinoid System in the Brain-Gut Axis," Gastroenterology 151, no. 2 (2016): 252–66; R. Pertwee, "Cannabinoids and the Gastrointestinal Tract." Gut 48, no. 6 (2001): 859–67.

48 Martin A. Lee, "CBD for Endurance Sports," Project CBD (February 21, 2020).

49 S. Engeli, "Dysregulation of the Endocannabinoid System in Obesity," Journal of Neuroendocrinology 20 (Suppl. 1): 110–15.

50 A. Dietrich and W.F. McDaniel, "Endocannabinoids and Exercise," British Journal of Sports Medicine 38, no. 5 (2004): 536–41.

51 Angie Hunt, "New Link Between Endocannabinoids and Exercise May Help in Treatment of Depression," Medical Xpress (August 14, 2009).

52 Paul Benhaim, "Will Hemp Replace Fish as the King of Omega-3?" NutraIngredients-Asia, updated February 6, 2020.

53 Martin A. Lee, "CBD & THC: Myths and Misconceptions," Project CBD, updated February 2, 2019.

54 J.M. Jamontt, A. Molleman, R.G. Pertwee, and M.E. Parsons, "The Effects of Δ9-tetrahydrocannabinol and Cannabidiol Alone and in Combination on Damage, Inflammation and In Vitro Motility Disturbances in Rat Colitis," British Journal of Pharmacology 160, no. 3 (June 2010): 712–23.

55 Sean D. McAllister, Liliana Soroceanu, and Pierre-Ives Desprez, "The Antitumor Activity of Plant-Derived Non-Psychoactive Cannabinoids," Journal of Neuroimmune Pharmacology 10, no. 2 (June 2015): 255–67.

56 John Merrick, Brian Lane, Terri Sebree, et al, "Identification of Psychoactive Degradants of Cannabidiol in Simulated Gastric and Physiological Fluid," Cannabis and Cannabinoid Research. 2016 ;1(1):102-112.

57 Franjo Grotenhermen, Ethan Russo, and Antonio Waldo Zuardi, "Even High Doses of Oral Cannabidiol Do Not Cause THC-Like Effects in Humans: Comment on Merrick et al. Cannabis and Cannabinoid Research 2016;1(1):102–12," Cannabis and Cannabinoid Research 2, no. 1 (January 1, 2017).

58 G. Nahler, F. Grotenhermen, A. Waldo Zuardi, and J.A.S. Crippa, "A Conversion of Oral Cannabidiol to Delta9-Tetrahydrocannabinol Seems Not to Occur in Humans," Cannabis and Cannibinoid Research 2, no. 1 (May 1, 2017): 81-86.

59 "2020 CBD Laws by State," CBD Awareness Project (January 13, 2020).

60 "Flying with CBD: What to Know About New TSA Airplane Rules," Travel Daily News (October 18, 2019).

61 Marcel O. Bonn-Miller, Mallory J.E. Loflin, and Brian F. Thomas et al., "Labeling Accuracy of Cannabidiol Extracts Sold Online," Journal of the American Medical Association 318, no. 17 (November 7, 2017): 1708–09.

Part II

1 Lisa L. Gill, "CBD Goes Mainstream," Consumer Reports (April 11, 2009).

2 "The Power of the Placebo Effect," Harvard Health Publishing, Harvard Medical School (May 2017), updated August 9, 2019.

3 Beth Israel Deaconess Medical Center, "Information as Important as Medication in Reducing Migraine Pain," ScienceDaily.

4 Adrian Devitt-Lee, "Cannabidiol and Epilepsy Meta-Analysis," Project CBD (November 7, 2018).

5 Judy George, "Cannabidiol Gets FDA Nod for New Indication," MedPage Today (August 3, 2020).

6 Melinda Misuraca, "Can CBD Help Your Complexion?" Project CBD (August 21, 2019).

7 Kinga Fanni Tóth, Dorottya Ádám, Tamás Bíró, and Attila Oláh, "Cannabinoid Signaling in the Skin: Therapeutic Potential of the 'C(ut)annabinoid' System," Molecules 24, no. 5 (2019): 918.

8 Ehrhardt Proksch, Michael Soeberdt, Claudia Neumann, Ana Kilic, and Christoph Abels, "Modulators of the Endocannabinoid System Influence Skin Barrier Repair, Epidermal Proliferation, Differentiation and Inflammation in a Mouse Model," Experimental Dermatology 28, no. 9 (September 2019): 1058–65.

9 Atila Oláh et al., "Cannabidiol Exerts Sebostatic and Antiinflammatory Effects on Human Sebocytes," Journal of Clinical Investigation 124, no. 9 (September 2, 2014): 3713–24.

10 B. Palmieri, C. Laurino, and M. Vadalà, "A Therapeutic Effect of CBD-Enriched Ointment in Inflammatory Skin Diseases and Cutaneous Scars," La Clinica terapeutica 170, no. 2 (March-April 2019): e93–e99.

11 Melinda Misuraca, "Bug Off: A True Story about CBD and MRSA," Project CBD (April 10, 2019).

NOTES

12 Giovanni Appendino et al., "Antibacterial Cannabinoids from Cannabis sativa: A Structure-Activity Study," Journal of Natural Products 71, no. 8 (August 6, 2008): 1427–30.

13 Melinda Misuraca, "Can CBD Help Your Complexion?" Project CBD (August 21, 2019).

14 Yasmin L. Hurd et al., "Early Phase in the Development of Cannabidiol as a Treatment for Addiction: Opioid Relapse Takes Initial Center Stage," Neurotherapeutics 12, no. 4 (October 2015): 807–15.

15 Adrian Devitt-Lee, "Drug Memories: CBD & Addiction," Project CBD (April 13, 2018).

16 Cristiane Ribeiro de Carvalho and Reinaldo Naoto Takahashi, "Cannabidiol Disrupts the Reconsolidation of Contextual Drug-Associated Memories in Wistar Rats," Addiction Biology 22, no. 3 (May 2017): 742–51.

17 Ibid.

18 Yanhua Ren, John Wittard, Alejandro Higuera-Mattas, Claudia V. Morris, and Yasmin L. Hurd, "Cannabidiol, a Nonpsychotropic Component of Cannabis, Inhibits Cue-Induces Heroin Seeking and Normalizes Discrete Mesolimbic Neuronal Disturbances," Journal of Neuroscience 29, no. 47 (November 25, 2009): 14764–69.

19 Adrian Devitt-Lee, "CBD & Opiate Addiction," Project CBD (May 29, 2019).

20 E. Fernández-Espejo and L. Núñez-Domínguez, "Endocannabinoid-Mediated Synaptic Plasticity and Substance Use Disorders," Neurología S0213-4853, no. 19 (March 8, 2019): 30010-6.

21 Francisco Alén et al., "Converging Action of Alcohol Consumption and Cannabinoid Receptor Activation on Adult Hippocampal Neurogenesis," International Journal of Neuropsychopharmacology 13, no. 2 (March 2010): 191–205.

22 Jack A. Prenderville, Áine M. Kelly, and Eric J. Downer, "The Role of Cannabinoids in Adult Neurogenesis," British Journal of Pharmacology 172, no. 16 (August 2015): 3950–63.

23 R. Andrew Chambers, "Adult Hippocampal Neurogenesis in the Pathogenesis of Addiction and Dual Diagnosis Disorders," Drug and Alcohol Dependence 130, no. 0 (June 1, 2013), 1–12.

24 "CBD Survey Results: Cultivating Wellness," Project CBD (2019).

25 Dustin Sulak, "America's Opiate Addiction Crisis and How Medical Canabis Can Help," Project CBD (August 2016).

26 "Summary of Key Findings," Project CBD.

27 Simon Haroutounian et al., "The Effect of Medicinal Canabis on Pain and Quality-of-Life Outcomes in Chronic Pain : A Prospective Open-Label Study," Clinical Journal of Pain 32, no. 12 (December 2016): 1036–43.

28 Dustin Sulak, "Cannabinoids in Harm Reduction: Physiology and Clinical Applications," NAADAC Annual Conference 2016.

29 Theresa Bennett, "CBD and COVID-19 Part 1: How Sales Are Trending," Cannabis Business Times (April 7, 2020).

30 Phoebe Luckhurst, "Could CBD Help Ease Your Covanxiety?" Evening Standard (April 27, 2020).

31 "Any Anxiety Disorder," National Institutes of Mental Health, updated November 2017. 10/14/20.

32 Alline C. Campos et al., "The Anxiolytic Effect of Cannabidiol on Chronically Stressed Mice Depends on Hippocampal Neurogenesis: Involvement of the Endocannabinoid System," International Journal of Neuropsychopharmacology 16, no. 6 (July 2013): 1407–19.

33 Mary Biles, "Cannabis, CBD & Anxiety," Project CBD (May 6, 2020).

34 Esther M. Blessing, Maria M. Steenkamp, Jorge Manzanares, and Charles R. Marmar, "Cannabidiol as a Potential Treatment for Anxiety Disorders," Neurotherapeutics 12, no. 4 (October 2015): 825–36.

35 José Alexandre Crippa et al., "Neural Basis of Anxiolytic Effects of Cannabidiol (CBD) in Generalized Social Anxiety Disorder: A Preliminary Report," Journal of Psychopharmacology 25, no. 1 (January 2011): 121–30.

36 Mateus M. Bergamaschi et al., "Cannabidiol Reduces the Anxiety Induced by Simulated Public Speaking in Treatment-Naïve Social Phobia Patients," Neuropsychopharmacology 36, no. 6 (May 2011): 1219–26.

37 "Summary of Key Findings," Project CBD.

38 Adrian Devitt-Lee, "CBD for the Morning Commute," Project CBD (October 29, 2019).

39 Ila M. Linares et al., "Cannabidiol Presents an Inverted U-Shaped Dose-Response Curve in a Simulated Public Speaking Test," Brazilian Journal of Psychiatry 41, no. 1 (January/February 2019).

40 Mary Biles, "Cannabis, CBD & Anxiety," Project CBD (May 6, 2020).
41 Alexandre Rafael de Mello Schier et al., "Cannabidiol, a Cannabis sativa Constituent, as an Anxiolytic Drug," Brazilian Journal of Psychiatry 34, suppl. 1 (June 2012): S104–10.
42 Stephen Schultz and Dario Siniscalco, "Endocannabinoid System Involvement in Autism Spectrum Disorder: An Overview with Potential Therapeutic Applications," AIMS Molecular Science 6, no. 1 (May 13, 2019): 27–37.
43 Dana Barchel et al., "Oral Cannabidiol Use in Children with Autism Spectrum Disorder to Treat Related Symptoms and Co-morbidities," Frontiers in Pharmacology 9 (January 9, 2019): 1521.
44 Lihi Bar-Lev Schleider et al., "Real Life Experience of Medical Canabis Treatment in Autism: Analysis of Safety and Efficacy," Nature.com (January 17, 2019).
45 Cannabis Conversations, "New Developments in Cannabid Medicine with Bonni Goldstein, MD," Project CBD, (March 9, 2020).
46 Natalya M. Kogan ct al., "Cannabidiol, a Major Non-Psychotropic Cannabis Constituent Enhances Fracture Healing and Stimulates Lysyl Hydroxylase Activity in Osteoblasts," Journal of Bone and Mineral Research 30, no. 10 (October 2015): 1905–13.
47 "Cancer Statistics," National Institutes of Health.
48 Martin A. Lee, "CBD, THC & Cancer," Project CBD (February 5, 2014).
49 Sean D. McAllister et al., "Pathways Mediating the Effects of Cannabidiol on the Reduction of Breast Cancer Cell Proliferation, Invasion, and Metastasis," Breast Cancer Research and Treatment 129, no. 1 (August 2011): 37–47.
50 Paula B. Dall'Stella et al., "Case Report: Clinical Outcome and Image Response of Two Patients with Secondary High-Grade Glioma Treated with Chemoradiation, PCV, and Cannabidiol," Frontiers in Oncology 8 (2016): 643.
51 Rudolf Likar, Markus Koestenberger, Martin Stultschnig, and Gerhard Nahler, "Concomitant Treatment of Malignant Brain Tumours with CBD—A Case Series and Review of the Literature," Anticancer Research 39, no. 10 (October 2019): 5797–5801.
52 Federation of American Societies for Experimental Biology, "CBD Shows Promise for Fighting Aggressive Brain Cancer," Newswise (April 27, 2020).
53 Patrícia Alves, Cristina Amaral, Natércia Teixeira, and Georgina Correia-da-Silva, "Cannabis sativa: Much More Beyond Δ9-tetrahydrocannabinol," Pharmacological Research 157 (July 2020): 104822.
54 G. Hu, G. Ren, and Y. Shi, "The Putative Cannabinoid Receptor GPR55 Promotes Cancer Cell Proliferation," Oncogene 30 (2011): 139–41.
55 Bandana Chakravarti, Janani Ravi, and Ramesh K. Ganju, "Cannabinoids as Therapeutic Agents in Cancer: Current Status and Future Implications," Oncotarget 5, no. 15 (August 2014): 5852–72
56 Barbara Romano et al., "Inhibition of Colon Carcinogenesis by a Standardized Cannabis sativa Extract with High Content of Cannabidiol," Phytomedicine 21, no. 5 (April 15, 2014): 631–39.
57 Sean D. McAllister, Liliana Soroceanu, and Pierre-Yves Desprez, "The Antitumor Activity of Plant-Derived Non-Psychoactive Cannabinoids," Journal of Neuroimmune Pharmacology 10, no. 2 (June 2015): 255–67.
58 Guillermo Velasco, Sonia Hernández-Tiedra, David Dávila, and Mar Lorente, "The Use of Cannabinoids as Anticancer Agents," Psychopharmacology and Biological Psychiatry 64 (January 4, 2016): 259–66.
59 Martin A. Lee, "CBD, THC & Cancer," Project CBD (February 5, 2014).
60 Cannabis Conversations, "New Developments in Cannabid Medicine with Bonni Goldstein, MD," Project CBD, (March 9, 2020).
61 Howard Meng et al., "Cannabis and Cannabinoids in Cancer Pain Management," Current Opinion in Supportive and Palliative Care 14, no. 2 (June 2020): 87–93
62 Ethan B. Russo, "Cannabinoids in the Management of Difficult to Treat Pain," Therapeutics and Clinical Risk Management 4, no. 1 (February 2008): 245–59.
63 Farjana Afrin et al., "Can Hemp Help? Low-THC Cannabis and Non-THC Cannabinoids for the Treatment of Cancer," Cancers 12, no. 4 (April 23, 2020): 1033.
64 "Marijuana and Cancer," American Cancer Society, last revised August 4, 2020.
65 Karen Getchell, "A Doctor's Advice: How to Use Cannabis During Chemotherapy," Leafly (July 2, 2019).

66 "Pain," Project CBD.

67 "Empower Doctors with Scientific Evidence for Medical Cannabis," PlantExt (March 11, 2019).

68 Ethan B. Russo, "Cannabinoids in the Management of Difficult to Treat Pain," Therapeutics and Clinical Risk Management 4, no. 1 (February 2008): 245–59.

69 Vijaya Iyer, "Sativex Relieves Pain in MS Patients, Italian Study Confirms," Multiple Sclerosis News Today (June 29, 2018).

70 Shelley Levitt, "CBD and Rheumatoid Arthritis: How It Worked for Me," The Healthy (February 5, 2020), last updated August 24, 2020.

71 McMaster University, "Cannabinoids vs. Placebo on Persistent Post-surgical Pain Following TKA: A Pilot RCT," ClinicalTrials.gov (February 1, 2019), last updated February 20, 2020.

72 Jason Socrates Bardi, "Turning Off Pain's Pathways," Scripps Research Institute News & Views 1, no. 22 (August 13, 2001).

73 Ethan Russo, "Clinical Endocannabinoid Deficiency and Genetic Regulation."

74 Danila De Gregorio et al., "Cannabidiol Modulates Serotonergic Transmission and Reverses Both Allodynia and Anxiety-Like Behavior in a Model of Neuropathic Pain," Pain 160, no. 1 (January 2019): 136–50.

75 Jacob M. Vigil et al., "The Therapeutic Effectiveness of Full Spectrum Hemp Oil Using a Chronic Neuropathic Pain Model," Life 10, no. 5 (May 18, 2020): 69.

76 "Arthritis Foundation Releases First CBD Guidance for Adults with Arthritis," Arthritis Foundation (September 24, 2019).

77 "CBD for Pain/CBD Survey Results: Cultivating Wellness," Project CBD.

78 "CBD for Arthritis Pain: What You Should Know," Arthritis Foundation.

79 Mary Biles, "Cannabis & the Immune System: A Complex Balancing Act," Project CBD (May 8, 2020).

80 Xixia Chu et al., "24-Hour-Restraint Stress Induces Long-Term Depressive-Like Phenotypes in Mice," Nature.com/Scientific Reports (September 9, 2016).

81 Dunleavy, Brian P., "Half of All Older Adults Are Worried about Dementia, Survey Says," United Press International.

82 Leonard Leinow and Juliana Birnbaum, "CBD as Preventative Medicine," Project CBD (November 7, 2017).

83 "Using CBD (Cannabidiol) to Treat the Symptoms of Alzheimer's & Other Dementias," Dementia Care Central (February 17, 2020).

84 Andras Bilkei-Gorzo, "The Endocannabinoid System in Normal and Pathological Brain Ageing," Philosophical Transactions of the Royal Society of London. Series B, Biological Sciences 367, no. 1607 (December 5, 2012): 3326–41.

85 G. Esposito et al., "Cannabidiol in vivo Blunts Beta-Amyloid Induced Neuroinflammation by Suppressing IL-1beta and iNOS Expression," British Journal of Pharmacology 151, no. 8 (August 2007): 1272–79.

86 "Using CBD (Cannabidiol) to Treat the Symptoms of Alzheimer's & Other Dementias," Dementia Care Central (February 17, 2020).

87 A. Vaarmann, S. Kovac, K.M. Holström, S. Gandhi, and A.Y. Abramov, "Dopamine Protects Neurons Against Glutamate-Induced Excitotoxicity," Cell Death & Disease 4, no. 1 (January 2013): e455.

88 María Rodríguez-Muñoz, Pilar Sánchez-Blázquez, Manuel Merlos, and Javier Garzón-Niño, "Endocannabinoid Control of Glutamate NMDA Receptors: The Therapeutic Potential and Consequences of Dysfunction," Oncotarget 7, no. 34 (August 23, 2016): 55840–62.

89 Georgia Watt and Tim Karl, "In vivo Evidence for Therapeutic Properties of Cannabidiol (CBD) for Alzheimer's Disease," Frontiers in Pharmacology 8 (2017): 20.

90 "Cannabinoids Remove Plaque-Forming Alzheimer's Proteins from Brain Cells," Salk.edu (June 27, 2016).

91 Maria Scherma et al., "New Perspectives on the Use of Cannabis in the Treatment of Psychiatric Disorders," Medicines 5, no. 4 (December 2018): 107.

92 Ethan Russo, "Introduction to the Endocannabinoid System," PHYTECS.com.

93 Matthew N. Hill et al., "Serum Endocannabinoid Content Is Altered in Females with Depressive Disorders: A Preliminary Report," Pharmacopsychiatry 41, no. 2 (March 2008): 48–53.

94 "Summary of Key Findings," Project CBD.

95 L. Weiss et al., "Cannabidiol Lowers Incidence of Diabetes in Non-Obese Diabetic Mice," Autoimmunity 39, no. 2 (March 2006): 143–51.

96 Abigail Klein Leichman, "Cannabis Extract to Be Used to Treat Diabetes," ISRAEL21c (April 21, 2015).

97 Prakash Nagarkatti et al., "Cannabinoids as Novel Anti-Inflammatory Drugs," Future Medicinal Chemistry 1, no. 7 (October 2009): 1333–49.

98 Jessica Caporuscio, "How Does Stress Affect Diabetes and Blood Sugar," Medical News Today (August 30, 2019).

99 Susan Lindeman, "CBD and Metformin—September 2020," cbdclinicals.com, updated September 9, 2020.

100 Jonathan Gotfried, Timna Naftali, and Ron Schey, "Role of Cannabis and Its Derivatives in Gastrointestinal and Hepatic Disease," Reviews in Basic and Clinical Gastroenterology and Hepatology 159 (2020): 62–80.

101 George Citroner, "Cannabis Oil May Reduce Symptoms for People with Crohn's Disease," Healthline (October 24, 2018).

102 Spink Health, "Cannabis Improves Symptoms of Crohn's Disease Despite Having No Effect on Gut Inflammation," EurekAlert! (October 21, 2018).

103 Martin A. Lee, ICRS 2018: Report from Leiden (Part 2), Project CBD (August 15, 2018).

104 Flavia Indrio et al., "Microbiota Involvement in the Gut–Brain Axis," Journal of Pediatric Gastroenterology and Nutrition 57 (December 2013): S11–S15.

105 Cannabis Conversation, "Dr. Ethan Russo: CBD, the Entourage Effect & the Microbiome," Project CBD (January 7, 2019).

106 Ibid.

107 Denise C Vidot et al., "Metabolic Syndrome Among Marijuana Users in the United States: An Analysis of National Health and Nutrition Examination Survey Data," American Journal of Medicine 129, no. 2 (February 2016): 173–39

108 Adrian Devitt-Lee, "CBD Extract for Ulcerative Colitis," Project CBD (May 28, 2019).

109 Peter M Irving et al., "A Randomized, Double-Blind, Placebo-Controlled, Parallel-Group, Pilot Study of Cannabidiol-Rich Botanical Extract in the Symptomatic Treatment of Ulcerative Colitis," Inflammatory Bowel Diseases 24, no. 4 (March 19, 2018): 714–24.

110 Chimezie Mbachi et.al, "Association Between Cannabis Use and Complications Related to Crohn's Disease: A Retrospective Cohort Study," Digestive Diseases and Sciences 64, no. 10 (October 2019): 2939–44.

111 Ibid.

112 Viola Brugnatelli et al. "Irritable Bowel Syndrome: Manipulating the Endocannabinoid System as First-Line Treatment," Frontiers in Neuroscience 14, no. 371 (April 21, 2020).

113 "Epilepsy & Seizure Facts," Epilepsy Foundation Michigan.

114 J M Cunha et al., "Chronic Administration of Cannabidiol to Healthy Volunteers and Epileptic Patients," Pharmacology 21, no. 3 (1980): 175–85.

115 Fabricio A. Pamplona, Lorenzo Rolim da Silva, and Ana Carolina Coan, "Potential Clinical Benefits of CBD-Rich Cannabis Extracts Over Purified CBD in Treatment-Resistant Epilepsy: Observational Data Meta-Analysis," Frontiers in Neurology 9 (September 12, 2018).

116 Adrian Devitt-Lee, "Cannabidiol & Epilepsy Meta-Analysis," Project CBD (November 7, 2018).

117 Ibid.

118 V. Giorgi et al., "Adding Medical Cannabis to Standard Analgesic Treatment for Fibromyalgia: A Prospective Observational Study," Clinical and Experimental Rheumatology 38, no. 1 (December 9, 2019): S53–S59.

119 Melinda Misuraca, "Cannabis & Chronic Fatigue Syndrome," Project CBD (December 11, 2019).

120 Ewa Kozela, Ana Juknat, and Zvi Vogel, "Modulation of Astrocyte Activity by Cannabidiol, a Nonpsychoactive Cannabinoid," International Journal of Molecular Sciences 18, no. 8 (July 31, 2017): 1669.

121 John F. Peppin and Robert B. Raffa, "The 'Missing Link' in the Physiology of Pain: Glial Cells," Practical Pain Management 16, no. 4 (updated May 18, 2016).

122 Mady Hornig et al., "Distinct Plasma Immune Signatures in ME/CFS Are Present Early in the Course of Illness," Science Advances 1, no. 1 (February 27, 2015).

123 "Heart Disease Facts," Centers for Disease Control and Prevention (September 8, 2020).

124 Makenzie L. Fulmer and Douglas P. Thewke, "The Endocannabinoid System and Heart Disease: The Role of Cannabinoid Receptor Type 2," Cardiovascular & Hematological Disorders Drug Targets 18, no. 1 (2018): 34–51.

125 Salahaden R. Sultan, Saoirse E. O'Sullivan, and Timothy J. England, "The Effects of Acute and Sustained Cannabidiol Dosing for Seven Days on the Haemodynamics in Healthy Men: A Randomised Controlled Trial," British Journal of Clinical Pharmacology 86, no. 6 (June 2020): 1125–38.

126 Khalid A. Jadoon, Garry D. Tan, and Saoirse E. O'Sullivan, "A Single Dose of Cannabidiol Reduces Blood Pressure in Healthy Volunteers in a Randomized Crossover Study," JCI Insight 2, no. 12 (June 15, 2017): e93760.

127 Martin A. Lee, "Project CBD Sunday: CBD Science Update," HeadyVermont (August 6, 2019).

128 Sarah K Walsh et. al., "Acute Administration of Cannabidiol In Vivo Suppresses Ischaemia-Induced Cardiac Arrhythmias and Reduces Infarct Size When Given at Reperfusion," British Journal of Clinical Pharmacology 160, no. 5 (July 2010): 1234–42.

129 Peter Grinspoon, "Cannabidiol (CBD): What We Know and What We Don't," Harvard Health Publishing, Harvard Medical School.

130 Ariane Mallat, Fatima Teixeira-Clerc, and Sophie Lotersztajn, "Cannabinoid Signaling and Liver Therapeutics," Journal of Hepatology 59, no. 4 (October 2013): 891–96.

131 Anna Parfieniuk and Robert Flisiak, "Role of Cannabinoids in Chronic Liver Diseases," World Journal of Gastroenterology 14, 40 (October 28, 2008): 6109–14.

132 Janice T. Chua et al., "Endocannabinoid System and the Kidneys: From Renal Physiology to Injury and Disease," Cannabis and Cannabinoid Research 4, no. 1 (March 13, 2019): 10–20.

133 Yuping Wang et al., "Cannabidiol Attenuates Alcohol-Induced Liver Steatosis, Metabolic Dysregulation, Inflammation and Neutrophil-Mediated Injury," Scientific Reports 7, no. 1, (September 21, 2017): 12064.

134 M.P. Lim, L.A. Devi, and R. Rozenfeld, "Cannabidiol Causes Activated Hepatic Stellate Cell Death Through a Mechanism of Endoplasmic Reticulum Stress-Induced Apoptosis," Cell Death & Disease 2, no. 6 (June 9, 2011): e170.

135 Lisa Rennie, "Can Using CBD Oil Cause Long-Term Damage to Your Liver," CBD Health & Wellness (November 22, 2018).

136 Bonni Goldstein, "Migraine Headaches [book excerpt]," Project CBD (January 17, 2017).

137 Ethan B. Russo, "Clinical Endocannabinoid Deficiency Reconsidered: Current Research Supports the Theory in Migraine, Fibromyalgia, Irritable Bowel, and Other Treatment-Resistant Syndromes," Cannabis and Cannabinoid Research 1, no. 1 (July 1, 2016): 154–65.

138 E. Russo, "Cannabis for Migraine Treatment: The Once and Future Prescription? An Historical and Scientific Review," Pain 76, no. 1-2 (May 1998): 3–8.

139 Lauren Pulling, "EAN 2017: Cannabinoids Suitable for Migraine Prophylaxis," Neuro Central (June 26, 2017).

140 Ibid.

141 Ethan B. Russo, "Clinical Endocannabinoid Deficiency Reconsidered: Current Research Supports the Theory in Migraine, Fibromyalgia, Irritable Bowel, and Other Treatment-Resistant Syndromes," Cannabis and Cannabinoid Research 1, no. 1 (2016): 154–165.

142 Stacey Kerr, "Managing Nausea with Cannabis," Hawaiian Ethos (February 2, 2018).

143 Irina Bancos, ed., "What Is Serotonin?" Hormone Health Network, updated December 2018.

144 James McIntosh, "What Is Serotonin and What Does It Do?," MedicalNewsToday (February 2, 2018).

145 Erin M. Rock et al., "Effect of Combined Oral Doses of Δ(9)-tetrahydrocannabinol (THC) and Cannabidiolic Acid (CBDA) on Acute and Anticipatory Nausea in Rat Models," Psychopharmacology 233, no. 18 (September 2016): 3353–60.

146 Erin M. Rock et al., "A Comparison of Cannabidiolic Acid with Other Treatments for Anticipatory Nausea Using a Rat Model of Contextually Elicited Conditioned Gaping," Psychopharmacology 231, no. 16 (August 2014): 3207–15.

147 Nishi Whiteley, "CBD & Parkinson's Disease," Project CBD (July 12, 2017).

148 "Non-Movement Symptoms," Parkinson's Foundation.

149 Christopher G. Goetz, "The History of Parkinson's Disease: Early Clinical Descriptions and Neurological Therapies," Cold Spring Harbor Perspectives in Medicine 1, no. 1 (September 2011): a008862.

150 Aidan J. Hampson, Julius Axelrod, and Maurizio Grimaldi, "Cannabinoids as Antioxidants and Neuroprotectants," US6630507B1, filed April 21, 1999, and issued October 7, 2003.

151 Alyssa S. Laun, "A study of GPR3, GPR6, of GPR12 as novel molecular targets for cannabidiol." (2018). Electronic Theses and Dissertations. Paper 2945.

152 Timothy R. Sampson et al., "Gut Microbiota Regulate Motor Deficits and Neuroinflammation in a Model of Parkinson's Disease," Cell 167,6 (December 1, 2016): 1469–80.e12.

153 Anastazja M. Gorecki et al., "Altered Gut Microbiome in Parkinson's Disease and the Influence of Lipopolysaccharide in a Human α-Synuclein Over-Expressing Mouse Model," Frontiers in Neuroscience 13 (August 7, 2019): 839.

154 Paula Perez-Pardo et al., "The Gut-Brain Axis in Parkinson's Disease: Possibilities for Food-Based Therapies," European Journal of Pharmacology 817 (December 15, 2017): 86–95.

155 Martin Lee, "Cannabinoid Science Sheds New Light on the Darkness of PTSD," MAPS Bulletin Annual Report (Winter 2013): 40–42.

156 Matthew N. Hill et al., "Reductions in Circulating Endocannabinoid Levels in Individuals with Post-Traumatic Stress Disorder Following Exposure to the World Trade Center Attacks," Psychoneuroendocrinology 38, no. 12 (September 10, 2013).

157 Rafael M. Bitencourt and Reinaldo N. Takahashi, "Cannabidiol as a Therapeutic Alternative for Post-Traumatic Stress Disorder: From Bench Research to Confirmation in Human Trials," Frontiers in Neuroscience 12 (July 24, 2018): 502.

158 Joan Oleck, "Cannabis May Help Veterans with PTSD. And Lawmakers May Be Acknowledging That," Forbes (March 30, 2020).159 Veterans Equal Access Act, H.R. 1647, 116th Cong. (in committee 3/12/2020).

160 F M Leweke et al., "Cannabidiol Enhances Anandamide Signaling and Alleviates Psychotic Symptoms of Schizophrenia," Translational Psychiatry 2, no. 3 (March 2012): e94.

161 Jonathan Knight, "Doping Down," New Scientist 2188 (May 29, 1999).

162 "New Insight into How Cannabidiol Takes Effect in the Brains of People with Psychosis," Science Daily (January 29, 2020).

163 Murat Yücel et al., "The Impact of Cannabis Use on Cognitive Functioning in Patients with Schizophrenia: A Meta-Analysis of Existing Findings and New Data in a First-Episode Sample," Schizophrenia Bulletin 38, no. 2 (March 2012): 316–30.

164 Harvey R. Colten and Bruce M. Altevogt, editors, Sleep Disorders and Sleep Deprivation: An Unmet Public Health Problem (Washington, DC: National Academies Press, 2006).

165 Lisa L Gill, "CBD Goes Mainstream," Consumer Reports (April 11, 2019).

166 "Summary of Key Findings: CBD Survey Results: Cultivating Wellness," Project CBD.

167 Ila M P Linares et al., "No Acute Effects of Cannabidiol on the Sleep-Wake Cycle of Healthy Subjects: A Randomized, Double-Blind, Placebo-Controlled, Crossover Study," Frontiers in Pharmacology 9 (April 5, 2018): 315.

168 Scott Shannon et al., "Cannabidiol in Anxiety and Sleep: A Large Case Series," Permanente Journal 23 (January 7, 2019): 18-041.

169 Charlotte Hilton Andersen, "How One Woman Used CBD Oil to Sleep Better and Beat Insomnia," The Healthy (May 18, 2020), last updated October 12, 2020.

170 Ethan B Russo et al., "Cannabis, Pain, and Sleep: Lessons from Therapeutic Clinical Trials of Sativex, a Cannabis-Based Medicine," Chemistry & Biodiversity 4, no. 8 (August 2007): 1729–43.

171 Kimberly A. Babson, James Sottile, and Danielle Morabito, "Cannabis, Cannabinoids, and Sleep: A Review of the Literature," Current Psychiatry Reports 19, no. 23 (March 27, 2017).

172 Simon Zhornitsky and Stéphane Potvin, "Cannabidiol in Humans—The Quest for Therapeutic Targets," Pharmaceuticals (Basel, Switzerland) 5, no. 5 (May 21, 2012): 529–52.

173 Anthony Nicholson et al. "Effect of Delta-9-tetrahydrocannabinol and Cannabidiol on Nocturnal Sleep and Early-Morning Behavior in Young Adults," Journal of Clinical Psychopharmacology 24, no. 3 (June 2004): 305–13.

174 Guoqiang Xing et al., "Differential Expression of Brain Cannabinoid Receptors Between Repeatedly Stressed Males and Females May Play a Role in Age and Gender-Related Difference in Traumatic Brain Injury: Implications from Animal Studies," Frontiers in Neurology 5 (August 28, 2014): 161.

175 "Traumatic Brain Injury in the United States: A Report to Congress," Prepared by: Division of Acute Care, Rehabilitation Research, and Disability Prevention, National Center for Injury Prevention and Control, Centers for Disease Control and Prevention, U.S. Department of Health and Human Services (December 1999).

176 Esther Shohami et al., "Endocannabinoids and Traumatic Brain Injury," British Journal of Pharmacology 163, no. 7 (August 2011): 1402–10.

177 Martin A. Lee, "No Brainer: CBD & THC for Head Injuries," Project CBD (May 2, 2018).

178 Tamsin Gregory and Martin Smith, "Cardiovascular Complications of Brain Injury," Continuing Education in Anaesthesia, Critical Care & Pain 12, no. 2 (April 2012): 67–71.

179 Sarah L. Walsh et al., "Acute Administration of Cannabidiol In Vivo Suppresses Ischaemia-Induced Cardiac Arrhythmias and Reduces Infarct Size When Given at Reperfusion," British Journal of Pharmacology 160, no. 5 (July 2010): 1234–42.

180 Chris Nickson, "Trauma Mortality and the Golden Hour," Life in the Fastlane (March 30, 2019).

181 Percival H. Pangilinan Jr. et al., "What Is the Pathophysiology of Secondary Traumatic Brain Injury (TBI)?" Medscape (March 2, 2020).

182 Martin A. Lee, "No Brainer: CBD & THC for Head Injuries," Project CBD (May 2, 2018).

183 Sarah L. Walsh et al. "Acute Administration of Cannabidiol In Vivo Suppresses Ischaemia-Induced Cardiac Arrhythmias and Reduces Infarct Size When Given at Reperfusion," British Journal of Pharmacology 160, no. 5 (July 2010): 1234–42.

184 William H. Hind, Timothy J. England, and Saiorse O'Sullivan, "Cannabidiol Protects an In Vitro Model of the Blood-Brain Barrier from Oxygen-Glucose Deprivation via PPARγ and 5-HT1A Receptors," British Journal of Pharmacology 173, no. 5 (March 2016): 815–25.

185 Ibid.

186 Martin A. Lee, "ICRS 2019: CBD for Anxiety, Cancer, Heart Disease, Addiction...," Project CBD (August 6, 2019).

187 Ethan B. Russo, "Cannabis Therapeutics and the Future of Neurology," Frontiers in Integrative Neuroscience 12 (October 18, 2018): 51.

188 Martin A. Lee, "ICRS 2018: Report from Leiden (Part 2)," Project CBD (August 15, 2018).

189 Jon Johnson, "Can CBD Help You Lose Weight?" MedicalNewsToday, (March 18, 2019).

190 Martin A. Lee, "Diet & the Endocannabinoid System," Project CBD, updated January 15, 2019.

191 Jonathan A Farrimond et al., "Cannabinol and Cannabidiol Exert Opposing Effects on Rat Feeding Patterns," Psychopharmacology 223, no. 1 (September 2012): 117–29.

192 Denise C. Vidot et al., "Metabolic Syndrome Among Marijuana Users in the United States: An Analysis of National Health and Nutrition Examination Survey Data," American Journal of Medicine 129, no. 2 (February 2016): 173–79.

193 Jonathan A Farrimond et al., "Cannabinol and Cannabidiol Exert Opposing Effects on Rat Feeding Patterns," Psychopharmacology 223, no. 1 (September 2012): 117–29.

194 Hilal Ahmad Parray and Jong Won Yun, "Cannabidiol Promotes Browning in 3T3-L1 Adipocytes," Molecular and Cellular Biochemistry 416 (April 11, 2016): 131–39.

195 Pál Pacher and George Kunos, "Modulating the Endocannabinoid System in Human Health and Disease: Successes and Failures," FEBS Journal 280, no. 9 (May 2013): 1918–43.

196 Bruce A. Watkins and Kim Jeffrey, "The Endocannabinoid System: Directing Eating Behavior and Macronutrient Metabolism," Frontiers in Psychology 5 (January 6, 2015).

197 Keane Lim et al., "A Systematic Review of the Effectiveness of Medical Cannabis for Psychiatric, Movement and Neurodegenerative Disorders," Clinical Psychopharmacology and Neuroscience 15, no. 4 (November 30, 2017): 301–12

198 "Summary of Key Findings: CBD Survey Results: Cultivating Wellness," Project CBD.

199 Jerome Bouaziz et al., "The Clinical Significance of Endocannabinoids in Endometriosis Pain Management," Cannabis and Cannabinoid Research 2, no. 1 (April 1, 2017): 72–80.

200 Terézia Kisková et al., "Future Aspects for Cannabinoids in Breast Cancer Therapy," International Journal of Molecular Sciences 20, no. 7 (April 3, 2019): 1673.

Part III

1 Renée Johnson, "Defining Hemp: A Fact Sheet," Congressional Research Service, updated March 19, 2019.

2 Martin A. Lee, "Cannabis Oil vs. Hemp Oil," Project CBD.

3 Ibid.

4 W. B. O'Shaughnessy, "On the Preparations of the Indian Hemp, or Gunjah: Cannabis Indica Their Effects on the Animal System in Health, and Their Utility in the Treatment of Tetanus and Other Convulsive Diseases," Provincial Medical Journal and Retrospect of the Medical Sciences 5, no. 123 (February 4, 1843): 363–69.

5 Zoe Sigman, "CBD Oil: An Introduction," Project CBD.

6 James Roland, "Is CBD a Safe and Effective Treatment for IBD and What's the Best Form to Use?" Healthline, updated on July 23, 2019.

7 Genevieve R. Moore, "How to Take Your CBD," Foria Wellness (September 30, 2019).

8 Marilyn A. Huestis, "Human Cannabinoid Pharmacokinetics," Chemistry & Biodiversity 4, no. 8 (August 2007): 1770–1804.

9 Lili Yang et al. "Cannabidiol Protects Liver from Binge Alcohol-Induced Steatosis by Mechanisms Including Inhibition of Oxidative Stress and Increase in Autophagy," Free Radical Biology & Medicine 68 (2014): 260–67.

10 Lisa L. Gill, "How to Safely Use CBD: Should You Inhale, Spray, Apply, or Eat It?" Consumer Reports (August 26, 2018).

11 Adrian Devitt-Lee, "What Is the Best Way to Take CBD?" Project CBD.

12 Jelena Grove, "Do Cannabis Suppositories Work?," Project CBD, updated January 14, 2020.

13 Yoshiteru Watanabe, "Permeation Pathways in Rectal Absorption: Anatomy and Physiology of the Rectum and Its Role in Drug Absorption," in Enhancement in Drug Delivery, ed. Elka Touitou and Brian W. Barry (Boca Raton, FL: Taylor & Francis Group, LLC, 2011), 136–38.

14 "Outbreak of Lung Injury Associated with the Use of E-Cigarette, or Vaping, Products," Centers for Disease Control and Prevention, updated February 25, 2020.

15 Mary Biles, "The CBD Silly Season," Project CBD, updated September 5, 2019.

16 D.C. Hammell et al., "Transdermal Cannabidiol Reduces Inflammation and Pain-Related Behaviours in a Rat Model of Arthritis," European Journal of Pain 20, no. 6 (July 2016): 936–48.

17 Marcel O. Bonn-Miller, Mallory J.E. Loflin, Brian F. Thomas et al., "Labeling Accuracy of Cannabidiol Extracts Sold Online," Journal of the American Medical Association 318, no. 17 (2017): 1708–9.

18 "How Do I Choose a CBD Product?" Project CBD, updated May 10, 2019.

19 Kathrin Klein and Ulrich M. Zanger, "Pharmacogenomics of Cytochrome P450 3A4: Recent Progress Toward the 'Missing Heritability' Problem," Frontiers in Genetics 4 (February 25, 2013): 12.

20 Ruth Gallily et al., "Overcoming the Bell-Shaped Dose-Response of Cannabidiol by Using Cannabis Extract Enriched in Cannabidiol," Pharmacology & Pharmacy 6, no. 2 (February 10, 2015): 75–85, doi:10.4236/pp.2015.62010.

21 Simon Zhornitsky and Stéphane Potvin, "Cannabidiol in Humans—The Quest for Therapeutic Targets," Pharmaceuticals (Basel) 5, no. 5 (May 21, 2012): 529–52.

22 "Dosing Guidelines from Mayo Clinic," Hawaii Cannabis Organization.

23 Martin A. Lee, "CBD & Cannabis Dosage Guide: Project CBD Interview with Dr. Sulak," Healer, updated April 1, 2019.

24 Harrison J. VanDolah, Brent A. Bauer, and Karen F. Mauck, "Clinicians' Guide to Cannabidiol and Hemp Oils," Mayo Clinic Proceedings 94, no. 9 (September 1, 2019): 1840–51.

25 Sophie A. Millar, Nicole L. Stone, Andrew S. Yates, and Saoirse E. O'Sullivan, "A Systematic Review on the Pharmacokinetics of Cannabidiol in Humans," Frontiers in Pharmacology 9 (November 26, 2018): 1365.

26 Julie Crockett, David Critchley, Bola Tayo, Joris Berwaerts, and Gilmour Morrison, "A Phase 1, Randomized, Pharmacokinetic Trial of the Effect of Different Meal Compositions, Whole Milk, and Alcohol on Cannabidiol Exposure and Safety in Healthy Subjects," Epilepsia, 61, no. 2 (February 2020): 267–77.

27 Irina Cherniakov, Dvora Izgelov, Abraham J Domb, and Amnon Hoffman, "The Effect of Pro Nano-Lipospheres (PNL) Formulation Containing Natural Absorption Enhancers on the Oral Bioavailability of Delta-9-tetrahydrocannabinol (THC) and Cannabidiol (CBD) in a Rat Model," European Journal of Pharmaceutical Sciences 109 (November 15, 2017): 21–30.

28 Jordan Tishler, "Inhaled vs. Oral Cannabis: Which Is Right for You?" green-flower.com (July 19, 2020).

29 Jahan Marcu, "How Safe Is Your Vape Pen?" Project CBD (July 14, 2015).

30 Kalpana S. Paudel, Dana C. Hammell, Remigius U. Agu, Satyanarayana Valiveti, and Audra L. Stinchcomb, "Cannabidiol Bioavailability After Nasal and Transdermal Application: Effect of Permeation Enhancers," Drug Development and Industrial Pharmacy, 36, no. 9 (September 2010): 1088–97.

31 Natascia Bruni et al., "Cannabinoid Delivery Systems for Pain and Inflammation Treatment," Molecules, 23, no. 10 (September 27, 2018): 2478.

32 "Cannabis Dosing: Dr. Dustin Sulak," Cannabis Conversations: Project CBD (May 23, 2016).

33 Judy George, "Benefits of CBD for Epilepsy Fades in One-Third of Patients: But the Observation That Two-Thirds Continued to Benefit May Be a Key Finding," MedPage Today, updated December 6, 2018.

34 Loren Devito, "Developing a Tolerance (or Reverse Tolerance) to CBD," CBD Health & Wellness Magazine (May 2, 2019).

35 Deepak Cyril D'Souza et al., "Rapid Changes in CB1 Receptor Availability in Cannabis Dependent Males After Abstinence from Cannabis," Biological Psychiatry: Cognitive Neuroscience and Neuroimaging 1, no. 1 (January 1, 2016): 60–7.

36 Harrison J. VanDolah, Brent A. Bauer, and Karen F. Mauck, "Clinicians' Guide to Cannabidiol and Hemp Oils," Mayo Clinic Proceedings 94: 9 (September 1, 2019): 1840–51.

37 World Health Organization, "Cannabidiol: Critical Review Report," Expert Committee on Drug Dependence, Fortieth Meeting, Geneva, June 4–7, 2018.

38 U.S. Food & Drug Administration, "What You Need to Know (And What We're Working to Find Out) About Products Containing Cannabis or Cannabis-Derived Compounds, Including CBD," www.fda.gov (March 5, 2020).

39 S.L. Dalterio and D.G. deRooij, "Maternal Cannabinoid Exposure. Effects on Spermatogenesis in Male Offspring," International Journal of Andrology 9, no. 4 (August 1986): 250–58.

40 Juan Pablo Prestifilippo et al., "Inhibition of Salivary Secretion by Activation of Cannabinoid Receptors," Experimental Biology and Medicine 231, no. 8 (September 2006): 1421–29.

41 "Category A: Health and Safety Risk," Project CBD.

42 Cannabis Conversations, "Cannabis Lab Testing & Safety Protocols," Project CBD (March 16, 2016).

43 Megan Brenan, "14% of Americans Say They Use CBD Products," Gallup (August 7, 2019).

44 Viola Brugnatelli, "It's Never Too Late to Start Using Medical Cannabis," Project CBD (November 18, 2019).

45 Ibid.

46 Cannabis Conversations, "Cannabis Therapeutics: Dr. Bonni Goldstein," Project CBD, (February 2, 2016).

47 Anna Symonds, "Cannabis for Contact Sports," Project CBD (July 24, 2019).

48 Bonni Goldstein, "Trade in Your Ibuprofen for Cannabis," Project CBD (May 6, 2019).

49 Oselys Rodriguez Justo et al., "Evaluation of in vitro Anti-Inflammatory Effects of Crude Ginger and Rosemary Extracts Obtained Through Supercritical CO_2 Extraction on Macrophage and Tumor Cell Line: The Influence of Vehicle Type," BMC Complementary Medicine and Therapies 15.

50 Monika Nagpal and Shaveta Sood, "Role of Curcumin in Systemic and Oral Health: An Overview," Journal of Natural Science, Biology and Medicine 4, no. 1 (January-June 2013): 3–7.

51 K. Prabhavathi et al., "A Randomized, Double Blind, Placebo Controlled, Cross Over Study to Evaluate the Analgesic Activity of Boswellia serrata in Healthy Volunteers Using Mechanical Pain Mode," Indian Journal of Pharmacology 46, no. 5 (September-October 2014): 475–79.

52 John N. Wood, "From Plant Extract to Molecular Panacea: A Commentary on Stone (1763) 'An Account of the Success of the Bark of the Willow in the Cure of the Agues,'" Philosophical Transactions of the Royal Society of London. Series B, Biological Sciences 370, no. 1666 (April 19, 2015): 20140317.

53 Kimberly A. Babson, James Sottile, and Danielle Morabito, "Cannabis, Cannabinoids, and Sleep: A Review of the Literature," Current Psychiatry Reports 19, no. 4 (April 2017): 23.

54 "Pet Parents Embrace CBD Products in Growing Pet Supplements Market," Packaged Facts (May 9, 2019).

55 Lauri-Jo Gamble et al., "Pharmacokinetics, Safety, and Clinical Efficacy of Cannabidiol Treatment in Osteoarthritic Dogs," Frontiers in Veterinary Science 5 (2018): 165.

56 Colorado State University, "CBD Clinical Trial Results on Seizure Frequency in Dogs 'Encouraging,'" EurekAlert! (May 21, 2019).

57 Kelly A. Deabold, Wayne S. Schwark, Lisa Wolf, and Joseph J. Wakshlag, "Single-Dose Pharmacokinetics and Preliminary Safety Assessment with Use of CBD-Rich Hemp Nutraceutical in Healthy Dogs and Cats," Animals 9, no. 10 (October 19, 2019): 832.

58 Ken Lambrecht, "What's the Latest on Using CBD for Pet Anxiety and Pain?" PetMD (October 31, 2018).

59 Lori Kogan, Regina Schoenfeld-Tacher, Peter Hellyer, and Mark Rishniw, "US Veterinarians' Knowledge, Experience, and Perception Regarding the Use of Cannabidiol for Canine Medical Conditions," Frontiers in Veterinary Science (January 10, 2019).

60 "What Drugs Will Interact with My Pet's CBD?" Blooming Culture (January 22, 2020).

Index